Post-Operative Rehabilitation Controversies in Athletes

Guest Editor

CLAUDE T. MOORMAN III, MD

CLINICS IN SPORTS MEDICINE

www.sportsmed.theclinics.com

Consulting Editor
MARK D. MILLER, MD

April 2010 • Volume 29 • Number 2

SAUNDERS an imprint of ELSEVIER, Inc.

W.B. SAUNDERS COMPANY

A Division of Elsevier Inc.

1600 John F. Kennedy Blvd. • Suite 1800 • Philadelphia, Pennsylvania 19103

http://www.theclinics.com

CLINICS IN SPORTS MEDICINE Volume 29, Number 2
April 2010 ISSN 0278-5919, ISBN-13: 978-1-4377-1874-4

Editor: Ruth Malwitz
Developmental Editor: Donald Mumford

Clinics in Sports Medicine (ISSN 0278-5919) is published quarterly by Elsevier Inc., 360 Park Avenue South, New York, NY 10010-1710. Months of issue are January, April, July, and October. Business and Editorial Offices: 1600 John F. Kennedy Blvd., Ste. 1800, Philadelphia, PA 19103-2899. Customer Service Office: 3251 Riverport Lane, Maryland Heights, MO 63043. Periodicals postage paid at New York, NY and additional mailing offices. Subscription prices are $278.00 per year (US individuals), $424.00 per year (US institutions), $140.00 per year (US students), $315.00 per year (Canadian individuals), $512.00 per year (Canadian institutions), $195.00 (Canadian students), $382.00 per year (foreign individuals), $512.00 per year (foreign institutions), and $195.00 per year (foreign students). Foreign air speed delivery is included in all *Clinics* subscription prices. All prices are subject to change without notice. **POSTMASTER:** Send address changes to *Clinics in Sports Medicine*, Elsevier Health Sciences Division, Subscription Customer Service, 3251 Riverport Lane, Maryland Heights, MO 63043. Customer Service (orders, claims, online, change of address): Elsevier Health Sciences Division, Subscription Customer Service, 3251 Riverport Lane, Maryland Heights, MO 63043. Tel: 1-800-654-2452 (U.S. and Canada); 314-447-8871 (outside U.S. and Canada). Fax: 314-447-8029. E-mail: journalscustomerservice-usa@elsevier.com (for print support); journalsonlinesupport-usa@elsevier.com (for online support).

Reprints. For copies of 100 or more of articles in this publication, please contact the Commercial Reprints Department, Elsevier Inc., 360 Park Avenue South, New York, NY 10010-1710. Tel.: 212-633-3812; Fax: 212-462-1935; E-mail: reprints@elsevier.com.

Clinics in Sports Medicine is covered in *MEDLINE/PubMed (Index Medicus) Current Contents/Clinical Medicine, Excerpta Medica,* and *ISI/Biomed.*

Printed and bound by CPI Group (UK) Ltd, Croydon, CR0 4YY

Transferred to Digital Print 2011

Contributors

CONSULTING EDITOR

MARK D. MILLER, MD
S. Ward Casscells Professor of Orthopaedic Surgery, University of Virginia, Charlottesville, Virginia; Team Physician, James Madison University, Harrisonburg, Virginia

GUEST EDITOR

CLAUDE T. MOORMAN III, MD
Director, Sports Medicine; Professor, Orthopaedic Surgery, Duke University School of Medicine, Durham, North Carolina

AUTHORS

KRISTOPHER J. AALDERINK, MD
Orthopaedic Surgery Sports Fellow, University of Iowa Sports Medicine Center, Department of Orthopaedic Surgery and Rehabilitation, University of Iowa Hospitals and Clinics, Iowa City, Iowa

ANNUNZIATO AMENDOLA, MD
Director of Division of Sports Medicine, University of Iowa Sports Medicine Center, Department of Orthopaedic Surgery and Rehabilitation, University of Iowa Hospitals and Clinics, Iowa City, Iowa

ROBERT B. ANDERSON, MD
Chief, Foot and Ankle Service; Vice Chief, Department of Orthopaedic Surgery, Carolinas Medical Center, OrthoCarolina, Charlotte, North Carolina

KAREN K. BRIGGS, MPH
Director, Department of Clinical Research, Steadman Philippon Research Institute, Vail, Colorado

STEPHEN S. BURKHART, MD
Clinical Associate Professor, Department of Orthopaedic Surgery, University of Texas Health Science Center at San Antonio, The San Antonio Orthopaedic Group, San Antonio, Texas

BRIAN J. COLE, MD, MBA
Professor, Cartilage Restoration Center, Division of Sports Medicine, Department of Orthopedic Surgery, Rush University Medical Center, Rush Medical College of Rush University, Chicago, Illinois

ANDREW J. COSGAREA, MD
Professor, Department of Orthopaedic Surgery, The Johns Hopkins University; Division Chief, Sports Medicine and Shoulder Surgery, The Johns Hopkins Hospital, Baltimore, Maryland

MARK P. COTE, PT, DPT
Sports Medicine Research Facilitator, Department of Orthopaedic Surgery, University of Connecticut Health Center, Farmington, Connecticut

KEELAN R. ENSEKI, MS, PT, ATC, OCS, SCS, CSCS
Centers for Rehab Services, Center for Sports Medicine; Department of Physical Therapy; Department of Sports Medicine and Nutrition, University of Pittsburgh, Pittsburgh, Pennsylvania

DONALD C. FITHIAN, MD
Southern California Permanente Medical Group, San Diego; Department of Orthopedic Surgery, Kaiser Permanente, El Cajon; Co-Director, San Diego Knee and Sports Medicine Fellowship, San Diego, California

GREGG GOMLINSKI, MSPT, CSCS
Senior Physical Therapist, Department of Rehabilitation Services, University of Connecticut Health Center, Farmington, Connecticut

GARY A. HORSMON, PA-C, ATC
Physician Assistant, Certified Athletic Trainer, Department of Orthopaedic Surgery, The Johns Hopkins University, Baltimore, Maryland

JASON M. HURST, MD
Joint Implant Surgeons, New Albany, Ohio

BRYAN T. KELLY, MD
Assistant Professor Orthopaedics, Hospital for Special Surgery, New York, New York

NAJEEB KHAN, MD
Fellow, San Diego Knee and Sports Medicine Fellowship, San Diego; Department of Orthopedic Surgery, Kaiser Permanente, El Cajon, California

SAMUEL S. KOO, MD, MPH
Shoulder Fellow, The San Antonio Orthopaedic Group, San Antonio, Texas

ROBROY MARTIN, PhD, PT, CSCS
Associate Professor, Department of Physical Therapy, Duquesne University; Staff Physical Therapist, Centers for Rehab Services, Center for Sports Medicine, University of Pittsburgh, Pittsburgh, Pennsylvania

AUGUSTUS D. MAZZOCCA, MS, MD
Associate Professor, Department of Orthopaedic Surgery, University of Connecticut Health Center, Farmington, Connecticut

JEREMY J. McCORMICK, MD
Assistant Professor of Orthopaedic Surgery, Department of Orthopaedic Surgery, Foot and Ankle Surgery, Washington University, Chesterfield, St Louis, Missouri

SHANE J. NHO, MD, MS
Assistant Professor, Cartilage Restoration Center, Division of Sports Medicine, Department of Orthopedic Surgery, Rush University Medical Center, Rush Medical College of Rush University, Chicago, Illinois

LUKE O'BRIEN, PT
Physical Therapist, Howard Head Sports Medicine Centers, Vail, Colorado

ROBERT A. PEDOWITZ, MD, PhD
Professor and Chair, UCLA/Orthopaedic Hospital, Department of Orthopedic Surgery, David Geffen School of Medicine at UCLA, Los Angeles, California

MICHAEL J. PENSAK, MD
Resident, Department of Orthopaedic Surgery, University of Connecticut, Medical Arts Building, Farmington, Connecticut

CHRISTOPHER M. POWERS, PhD, PT
Co-Director, Musculoskeletal Biomechanics Research Laboratory; Director, Program in Biokinesiology, Division of Biokinesiology and Physical Therapy; Professor of Biokinesiology and Physical Therapy, University of Southern California, Los Angeles, California

WILLIAM G. RODKEY, DVM, Diplomate ACVS
Chief Scientific Officer, Steadman Philippon Research Institute, Vail, Colorado

JESSICA H.J. RYU
Tulane Medical School, New Orleans, Louisiana

NIMA SALARI, MD
Resident, Department of Orthopaedic Surgery, The Johns Hopkins University, Baltimore, Maryland

DANIEL A. SEIGERMAN, MD
Resident, Department of Orthopaedic Surgery, New Jersey Medical School, University of Medicine and Dentistry of New Jersey, Newark, New Jersey

MICHAEL SHAFFER, PT, ATC, OCS
Coordinator for Sports Rehabilitation, University of Iowa Sports Medicine Center, Department of Orthopaedic Surgery and Rehabilitation, University of Iowa Sports Medicine, Iowa City, Iowa

J. RICHARD STEADMAN, MD
Orthopaedic Surgeon and Principal, Steadman-Hawkins Clinic; Founder and Chairman, Steadman Philippon Research Institute, Vail, Colorado

KAREN E. WOJCIK, MSPT, ATC
Senior Physical Therapist, Department of Rehabilitation Services, University of Connecticut Health Center, Farmington, Connecticut

Contents

Foreword **xi**

Mark D. Miller

Preface **xiii**

Claude T. Moorman III

Rehabilitation Following Arthroscopic Rotator Cuff Repair **203**

Samuel S. Koo and Stephen S. Burkhart

The postoperative rehabilitation program is critical for the successful arthroscopic treatment of rotator cuff injury. The authors' experience has confirmed that the best clinical results (restoration of strength, motion, and relief of pain) following rotator cuff repair are achieved after a durable repair of tendon to bone that heals in its entirety. Therefore, the senior author (S.S.B.) has adopted a customized rehabilitation protocol to optimize postoperative range of motion while maintaining rotator cuff integrity. A customized rehabilitation program that begins closed-chained overhead stretches (table slides) early for groups at risk for developing stiffness and delays overhead stretches for the remaining patients until 6 weeks is best to avoid stiffness without potentially increasing the risk of rerupture in the early postoperative period.

Rehabilitation of Acromioclavicular Joint Separations: Operative and Nonoperative Considerations **213**

Mark P. Cote, Karen E. Wojcik, Gregg Gomlinski, and Augustus D. Mazzocca

Acromioclavicular joint (AC) separations are one of the most common injuries seen in orthopedic and sports medicine practices, accounting for 9% of all injuries to the shoulder girdle. Various operative and nonoperative treatment schemes have been described for the management of AC joint injuries. Although there is controversy about the efficacy of surgical reconstruction versus nonoperative intervention for grade III type injuries, grade I and II separations seem to respond favorably to conservative management. Conversely, grades IV, V, and VI often require surgical reconstruction. Regardless of the type of injury, rehabilitation as a part of conservative management and postoperative care plays an important role in the management of these injuries. This article presents a rehabilitation approach to treatment of acromioclavicular separations pre- and postoperatively.

Rehabilitation of Biceps Tendon Disorders in Athletes **229**

Jessica H.J. Ryu and Robert A. Pedowitz

The diagnosis and management of an active patient with biceps disease can be challenging for the treating physician. A careful review of the function, anatomy, and pathology of biceps in conjunction with a thorough, knowledgeable history and physical examination can yield a working diagnosis in this challenging patient population. The physician must also be aware of the physiology of postsurgical repair and advocate appropriate rehabilitation activities that correlate with the timeline of secure tissue healing. This article focuses on nonsurgical rehabilitation and postoperative rehabilitation of biceps tendon injuries.

Rehabilitation After Arthroscopic Decompression for Femoroacetabular Impingement **247**

Keelan R. Enseki, RobRoy Martin, and Bryan T. Kelly

The use of arthroscopic technology to address pathologic conditions of the hip joint has become a topic of growing interest in the orthopedic community. Addressing femoroacetabular impingement through this method has generated additional attention. As surgical options evolve, rehabilitation protocols must meet the challenge of providing a safe avenue of recovery, yet meeting the goal of returning to high levels of functioning. Current rehabilitation concepts should be based on the growing body of evidence, knowledge of tissue healing properties, and clinical experience.

Rehabilitation Following Microfracture for Chondral Injury in the Knee **257**

Jason M. Hurst, J. Richard Steadman, Luke O'Brien, William Rodkey, and Karen K. Briggs

Full-thickness chondral defects in the knee are common, and these articular cartilage lesions may present in various clinical settings and at different ages. Articular cartilage defects that extend full thickness to subchondral bone rarely - by providing a suitable environment for new tissue formation and takes advantage of the body's own healing potential. Proper surgical technique and rehabilitation improve the success rate of the microfracture procedure. The goals are to alleviate the pain and disability that can result from chondral lesions and restore joint conformity, thereby preventing late degenerative changes in the joint.

Rehabilitation After Autologous Chondrocyte Implantation in Athletes **267**

Shane J. Nho, Michael J. Pensak, Daniel A. Seigerman, and Brian J. Cole

Over the years a variety of cartilage restorative procedures have been developed for athletes to address focal, full-thickness cartilaginous defects in the knee joint, including microfracture, osteochondral autografts, osteochondral allografts, autologous chondrocyte implantation (ACI), and most recently, next-generation ACI involving scaffolds or cell-seeded scaffolds. Since its introduction, ACI has yielded some very promising results in athletes and nonathletes alike. Rehabilitation following ACI requires an in-depth understanding of joint mechanics, and knowledge of the biologic and biomechanical properties of healing articular cartilage. A patient-, lesion-, and sports-specific approach is required on the part of the trainer or physical therapist to gradually restore knee joint function and strength so that the athlete may be able to return to competitive play. This article reviews the rehabilitation protocols for injured athletes following an ACI procedure.

Foreword

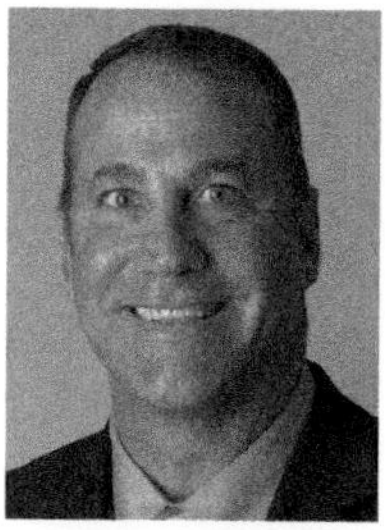

Mark D. Miller, MD
Consulting Editor

As an orthopedic surgeon, rehabilitation is one of my least favorite topics! Nevertheless, it is a very important part of surgical success. So it is essential that I (and all of us) pay attention. To give us some insight on this important topic, Dr Moorman (known fondly as "T" to most of us) has put together an all-star team of surgeons to outline the rehabilitation protocols related to the procedures for which the surgeons are best known. T has done an outstanding job in this as in everything he does! Many important orthopedic procedures are included, but the focus is on the knee and shoulder. I would suggest that, as painful as it might be, we all go through this issue with our rehabilitation protocols and red pen in hand, and listen to some expert advise. That's what I'm doing.

Mark D. Miller, MD
S. Ward Casscells Professor of Orthopaedic Surgery
Department of Orthopaedic Surgery
University of Virginia
400 Ray C. Hunt Drive, Suite 330
Charlottesville, VA 22908-0159, USA

E-mail address:
mdm3p@virginia.edu

Clin Sports Med 29 (2010) xi
doi:10.1016/j.csm.2010.01.001
sportsmed.theclinics.com

Preface

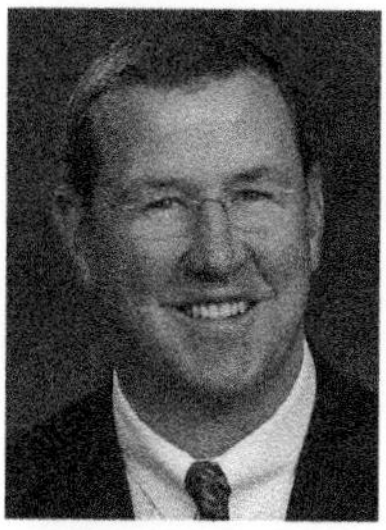

Claude T. Moorman III, MD
Guest Editor

Rehabilitation following many sports medicine operative procedures has received much less emphasis than the technical aspects of surgery. Often the approach in protocol for postoperative management is arbitrary and unproven. The data-driven approach most of us have adopted using leveled evidence has not been available. I do not expect to entirely rectify this in the current issue of the *Clinics in Sports Medicine*, but hope to provide directed "inside information" by topic from the best experts available. The format of this issue will be to structure these recommended protocols around a "Top Ten" list of procedures whose optimal rehabilitation has advanced or remains controversial. These procedures cover the anatomy from the toe to the top of the shoulder for the athlete. I believe this compendium of excellent articles will provide invaluable adjuncts to the busy sports medicine surgeon and those currently in training. I am tremendously indebted to the contributors who have been chosen as the top authority in their particular areas.

Godspeed!

Claude T. Moorman III, MD
Duke University School of Medicine
Box 3639 DUMC
Durham, NC 27710, USA

E-mail address:
moorm001@mc.duke.edu

Clin Sports Med 29 (2010) xiii
doi:10.1016/j.csm.2009.12.011

Rehabilitation Following Arthroscopic Rotator Cuff Repair

Samuel S. Koo, MD, MPH[a], Stephen S. Burkhart, MD[b,*]

KEYWORDS

• Stiffness • Postoperative stiffness • Complications
• Rotator cuff • Rotator cuff repair • Physical therapy
• Arthroscopic shoulder surgery

The postoperative rehabilitation program is critical to the success of surgical treatment of rotator cuff injury. Numerous rehabilitation protocols for the management of rotator cuff disease exist and are primarily based on anecdotal clinical observation. Millett and colleagues[1] described a commonly used rehabilitation protocol consisting of passive range of motion for the first 6 weeks followed by active range of motion starting in the seventh postoperative week. The rationale for the prescribed rehabilitation protocol was based on "empiric clinical experience." Stiffness is the most common complication after rotator cuff repair, independent of repair technique.[2] As a result, many surgeons start aggressive rehabilitation early to prevent postoperative stiffness. However, multiple clinical studies show that early motion may result in devastating consequences. For example, in the presence of rotator cuff muscle atrophy, a 25% to 94% chance of recurrent cuff tear has been reported.[3,4] Results obtained after revision rotator cuff repairs are inferior to those of primary repairs.[5] Therefore, it is imperative to avoid the temptation of beginning motion or strengthening too early to limit the number of re-tears that occur. In the authors' experience, stiffness is a complication that is much easier to overcome than recurrent cuff tears. Furthermore, the literature has shown that treatment for postoperative stiffness is effective and satisfactory to the patient.[6,7] Arthroscopic lysis of adhesions and capsular release are reliable in restoring the range of motion for those patients who develop clinically significant postoperative stiffness after rotator cuff repair.[6,7]

Disclosure: Dr Burkhart is a Consultant for Arthrex.

[a] The San Antonio Orthopaedic Group, 150 East Sonterra Boulevard, Suite 300, San Antonio, TX 78258, USA

[b] Department of Orthopaedic Surgery, University of Texas Health Science Center at San Antonio, The San Antonio Orthopaedic Group, 150 East Sonterra Boulevard, Suite 300, San Antonio, TX 78258, USA

* Corresponding author.

E-mail address: ssburkhart@msn.com (S.S. Burkhart).

Clin Sports Med 29 (2010) 203–211
doi:10.1016/j.csm.2009.12.001
sportsmed.theclinics.com

CUSTOMIZED REHABILITATION

A rehabilitation program that best allows for tendon to bone healing while preventing shoulder stiffness has not definitively been established. This is a matter that requires careful judgment because an overly conservative approach tends to promote stiffness, whereas an overly aggressive tactic can result in recurrent tears. The best clinical results (restoration of strength, motion, and relief of pain) after rotator cuff repair are achieved with the use of a customized rehabilitation protocol to optimize postoperative range of motion while maintaining rotator cuff integrity.

After repair of large to massive rotator cuff tears (tears greater than 5 cm or involvement of more than 2 tendons), the authors have adopted a conservative rehabilitation protocol (**Box 1**). Because of the precarious nature of these repairs, with reported retear rates as high as 94%,[3] this rehabilitation protocol avoids potentially destructive high strains at the repair site in the early postoperative period[8,9] and encourages more parallel collagen orientation and improved mechanical properties in the healed rotator cuff.[10] In addition, by delaying strengthening until postoperative 3 to 4 months, the conservative protocol allows Sharpey fibers to form before stressing the repair with resistive exercises (as previously shown in primates).[11] Thus, the conservative rehabilitation protocol is recommended for patients with large to massive tears.

Some patients who have undergone rotator cuff surgery have a higher-than-average risk for the development of postoperative stiffness. This group includes patients with coexisting calcific tendinitis, adhesive capsulitis, partial articular supraspinatus tendon avulsion (PASTA)-type rotator cuff repair, concomitant labral repair, and single-tendon rotator cuff repair.[6] For these patients, a modified, more accelerated rehabilitation program is used (**Box 2**). The patients in this group begin closed-chained overhead motion (table slides) immediately after the surgery (**Fig. 1**). These patients can tolerate the small additional strain at the repair site without increasing the incidence of recurrent tears.[6] Early closed-chained overhead motionhelps keep the rate of stiffness quite low in this high-risk group of patients (less than 1%). For patients who fall into the high-risk category, the authors institute the accelerated rehabilitation protocol.

UNDERSTANDING POSTOPERATIVE STIFFNESS

Much of the protocol described in this article is based on the authors' data on postoperative stiffness after arthroscopic rotator cuff repair. A review of the literature reveals that the rate of postoperative stiffness after rotator cuff repair is from 0% to 14%.[12–15] The authors used a conservative rehabilitation protocol for all their patients with arthroscopic rotator cuff repair, and their data showed a comparable overall rate (4.9%) of postoperative adhesion formation and motion restriction requiring a secondary arthroscopic release.[6] However, certain risk factors associated with an increased prevalence of stiffness were identified among patients positive for selected risk factors. In the study, the development of clinically significant stiffness requiring arthroscopic capsular release and lysis of adhesions was more prevalent in patients with rotator cuff repair who had coexisting calcific tendonitis (16.7%), adhesive capsulitis (15%), PASTA-type rotator cuff repair (13.5%), concomitant labral repair (11%), or single-tendon rotator cuff repair (7.3%).[6] A total of 231 of 489 patients undergoing arthroscopic rotator cuff repair were positive for at least 1of these conditions, and 18 (7.8%) of these patients developed stiffness, whereas only 6 (2.3%) of 258 patients negative for all of these risk factors developed stiffness. As a result of this study, the authors have elected to treat all patients with rotator cuff repair who are not a part of the high-risk patient group with the conservative rehabilitation protocol.

Box 1
Rehabilitation protocol following arthroscopic repair of massive rotator cuff tears

Preoperative period

Surgeon-directed counseling on rehabilitation plan

Give patient therapy kit and instruct on initial use

Therapy kit: polyvinyl chloride (PVC) cane, rope and pulley, and graduated elastic strengthening bands

Immediate postoperative period

Patient's arm placed in sling with small pillow (Ultra-Sling; DJ Ortho, Carlsbad, CA, USA)

Surgeon gives patient and family specifics of rehabilitation plan

Postoperative weeks 0 to 6

Postoperative day 1 to 10 at initial follow-up, surgeon-directed reinforcement of home rehabilitation plan

Remove sling 3 times per day for

- Active motion of hand, wrist, and elbow
- Passive external rotation of shoulder with arm at side (use PVC cane)
  - Limited to 0° (straight ahead) for massive tears and subscapularis tears
- No active assisted motion

Postoperative weeks 7 to 16

Discontinuation of sling and continuation of previous exercises

- Advance passive external rotation with cane (limit at external rotation of opposite shoulder)
- Start table slides and rope and pulley overhead stretch
- Still No active assisted motion
- No strengthening

Postoperative months 4 to 6

Continue previous stretching exercises

- Add internal rotation stretches

Begin strengthening program with graduated elastic bands

- Internal and external rotation with arm at side (deltoid and rotator cuff)
- Curl and low row exercise (biceps and periscapular muscles)
- No heavy overhead lifting and no acceleration of arm in sport

Patient is given option of using therapist to assist in implementation of our plan

Postoperative months 6 to 12

May progress to using light weights in gym

Massive cuff tear patients continue overhead lifting restriction and sport restriction until 1 year

A second study was conducted using a customized rehabilitation protocol based on risk factors for stiffness. This study showed that the prevalence of postoperative stiffness was reduced dramatically in the high-risk patient group in comparison to the earlier study. The purpose of the second study was to determine the benefits of

Box 2
Modified rehabilitation protocol following arthroscopic rotator cuff repair for patients at high risk for stiffness

Preoperative period

Surgeon-directed counseling on rehabilitation plan

Give patient therapy kit and instruct on initial use

Therapy kit: PVC cane, rope and pulley, and graduated elastic strengthening bands

Immediate postoperative period

Patient's arm placed in sling with small pillow

Surgeon gives patient and family specifics of rehabilitation plan

Postoperative weeks 0 to 6

Postoperative day 1 to 10 at initial follow-up, surgeon-directed reinforcement of home rehabilitation plan

Remove sling 3 times per day for

- Active motion of hand, wrist, and elbow
- Passive external rotation of shoulder with arm at side (use PVC cane)
    - Limited to 0° (straight ahead) for subscapularis tears
- No active assisted motion
- Table slides for passive overhead motion

Postoperative weeks 7 to 12

Discontinuation of sling and continuation of previous exercises

- Advance passive external rotation with cane (limit at external rotation of opposite shoulder)
- Continue with table slides and add rope and pulley overhead stretch
- No strengthening

Postoperative months 3 to 6

Continue previous stretching exercises

- Add internal rotation stretches

Begin strengthening program with graduated elastic bands

- Resisted internal and external rotation with arm at side (deltoid and rotator cuff)
- Curl and low row exercise (biceps and periscapular muscles)
- No heavy overhead lifting and no acceleration of arm in sport

Patient is given option of using therapist to assist in implementation of plan

Postoperative months 6 to 12

May progress to using light weights in gym

Clearance to full activity given based on examination, typically at 6 months

a modified, accelerated physical therapy protocol in reducing the prevalence of postoperative stiffness after arthroscopic rotator cuff repair for patients having at least 1 of the 5 risk factors mentioned earlier. During the 17-month study period from September 2006 to January 2008, the senior author (SSB) performed 198 arthroscopic rotator cuff

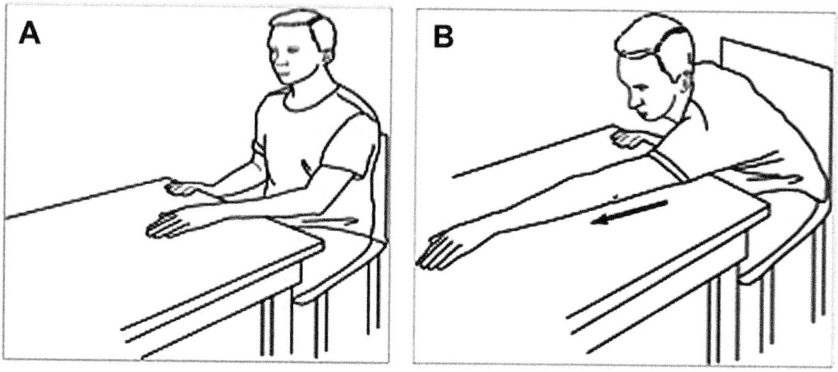

Fig. 1. (*A, B*) Table slides. Seated at a table, place the hand of the affected shoulder on a sliding surface (ie, place hand on a magazine that slides against a smooth table surface). Place the opposite (unaffected) hand on the wrist of the affected side to initiate and stabilize the motion. Slowly slide the affected hand along the table and bring the head down toward the surface of the table until shoulder is in an elevated position relative to the head. Hold the stretch for 15 to 20 seconds and repeat 10 times. Patients repeat this exercise 2 to 3 times daily.

repairs in 192 patients. These patients were prospectively assigned to either a conservative or a modified rehabilitation program, depending on the presence of any of the 5 risk factors. The conservative program prescribed immediate passive external rotation, but patients did not begin overhead stretches or table slides until 6 weeks postoperation. The modified program prescribed immediate table slides for passive overhead motion, and, in the absence of a subscapularis tear, passive external rotation.

Among the 192 patients, 105 were assigned to the conservative rehabilitation protocol and 87, who were identified as belonging to the high-risk group, were started on the modified protocol. One of the 105 patients who underwent conservative therapy developed postoperative stiffness, a prevalence that was not significantly different from the 2.3% prevalence from the previous study (P = .350), and 88 (84%) had complete follow-up visit data collected at a median of 8 months, with a range of 2 to 25 months. Among the 87 patients assigned to the modified protocol, the positive counts for selected risk factors were as follows: (1) 6 had adhesive capsulitis, (2) 6 had calcific tendinitis, (3) 11 had concomitant labral repair, (4) 18 had PASTA-type rotator cuff tear, (5) and 79 had single-tendon rotator cuff tear. Twenty-six patients were positive for more than one risk factor. None of these patients developed postoperative stiffness, which was a significantly lower prevalence than the 7.8% prevalence from the previous study (P = .003). Complete follow-up data were available for all 87 patients, with median follow-up of 9 months and a range of 2 to 23 months. Taken as a whole, the single case of postoperative stiffness out of 198 repairs defined an overall prevalence that was significantly lower than the 4.9% prevalence reported for the previous study (P = .002).

An equally important factor in determining the extent of rehabilitation is the potential treatment for complications that may occur after repair. Stiffness is the most common complication after rotator cuff repair but is easily treatable. All 24 patients with clinically significant stiffness requiring arthroscopic lysis of adhesions and capsular release regained their motion after the second surgery (median of 32 month follow-up). Furthermore, at the time of second-look arthroscopy, 23 of the 24 patients had complete healing of the original pathology. One patient had a defect remaining in the rotator cuff, with healing of 60% of the repaired footprint. All patients were satisfied with the eventual outcome. Therefore, secondary surgery for postoperative stiffness is reliable. On the other hand, if a patient experiences a recurrent tear that requires a second repair, the result of the revision surgery is far less predictable.

As a direct result of these studies, the senior author (SSB) divides the postoperative rehabilitation after rotator cuff repairs into 2 categories. In the first group, patients identified as being at high risk for postoperative stiffness (rotator cuff repairs with coexisting calcific tendonitis, adhesive capsulitis, PASTA-type rotator cuff repair, concomitant labral repair, and single-tendon rotator cuff repair) are started on the accelerated modified rehabilitation protocol. The second group, which includes all other patients that do not fit into the high-risk category, are started on the conservative rehabilitation protocol.

The results obtained show that a rehabilitation program that begins closed-chained overhead stretches (table slides) early for groups at risk for developing stiffness is best to avoid stiffness without potentially increasing the risk for rerupture in the early post-operative period. Furthermore, limiting potentially destructive stresses at the repair site for patients without increased risk for postoperative stiffness helps to promote healthy healing without unduly compromising the integrity of the rotator cuff repair.

THE REHABILITATION PHILOSOPHY

Effective communication and coordination of care by the physical therapist and shoulder surgeon are essential in optimal patient outcomes after rotator cuff repair. In the ideal situation, a well-educated therapist who has great communication with the treating surgeon can customize the therapy for each patient and mobilize the shoulder early, reestablish scapulothoracic function, and minimize the risk of stiffness and re-tear, while facilitating return to function. However, this ideal situation is often not attainable. In practice, the patient is encouraged to take responsibility for the first portion of the rehabilitation. For the most part, if the patient is agreeable, rehabilitation during the first 3 months, which consists mostly of stretching, is conducted entirely by the patient. In this way, therapy visits are reserved for the more difficult task of regaining strength, beginning in the third and fourth postoperative months. The authors have found this method to work well with their patients.

THE REHABILITATION PROTOCOL

The authors suggest using a customized rehabilitation protocol dependent on rotator cuff tear size and the presence of clinical risk factors for stiffness.

Immediate Postoperative Period to 6 Weeks

All patients

All patients who undergo arthroscopic rotator cuff repair are instructed to perform elbow range of motion exercises starting the day after surgery. In addition, if the subscapularis was not involved in the repair, patients also begin passive external rotation to an extent that can be tolerated by them. If the subscapularis has been repaired, passive external rotation beyond 0° is prohibited. Typically, patients are encouraged to remove the shoulder sling at least 3 to 4 times a day, once for each meal and again when taking a shower. A shoulder sling is worn for the first 6 weeks. All patients are given a customized therapy kit that allows them to perform the necessary exercises at home without going to a therapist.

High-risk patients
During the first 6 postoperative weeks, patients at high risk for developing shoulder stiffness are instructed to begin an accelerated shoulder rehabilitation program.[6] This entails starting closed-chain, passive overhead range of motion exercises (ie, table slides) (see **Fig. 1**) and passive external rotation exercises (for those without subscapularis repairs) during the first 6 weeks. Each patient receives a therapy kit and typically manages the individual stretching program after being instructed in the clinic.

Lower-risk patients
All other patients who undergo rotator cuff repair begin only passive external rotation exercises (for those without subscapularis repairs) and not overhead table slides until 6 weeks postoperation. All patients continue with the elbow range of motion exercises.

Postoperative 7th to 12th Weeks

Beginning in the 7th and progressing to the 12th postoperative week, all patients are instructed to perform passive overhead stretches with a rope and pulley. During this period, patients continue with elbow range of motion and passive external rotation exercises. No strengthening is allowed at this time. This is the same for high-risk and non–high-risk patients.

Postoperative Third to Fourth Months

At 3 to 4 months postoperation, patients begin strengthening exercises with elastic bands. The exact time to start strengthening depends primarily on rotator cuff tear size. In patients with massive tears, defined as rotator cuff tear size greater than 5 cm or involvement of 2 or more tendons, strengthening is delayed until 4 months postoperation. Furthermore, patients with revision cuff repair do not begin strengthening until 4 months. All other patients may begin strengthening at 3 months. The strengthening consists of the "four pack," which includes resisted external and internal rotation, biceps curls, and a low row exercise (to strengthen the scapular stabilizers).

Postoperative 4 Months to 1 Year

During the first 6 postoperative months, patients are restricted from performing heavy overhead lifting and aggressive activity that requires acceleration of the arm (golf, tennis, overhand throw). Patients are then typically allowed to return to unlimited activities at 6 months postoperation, with the exception of patients with massive 3-tendon tear and patients who underwent revision repair; these patients are allowed full activities at 1 year. Activities that accelerate the arm in space (ie, golf swing, tennis) are especially to be avoided until the full 6 months for patients with smaller cuff tears and until 1 year for patients with massive cuff tears.

ARTHROSCOPIC ROTATOR CUFF REPAIR

Given the conservative nature of the rehabilitation protocol, an increased incidence of postoperative stiffness might be expected. This is particularly true for large and massive rotator cuff tears, where passive motion is delayed until postoperative sixth week, and strengthening until postoperative fourth month. This is a reasonable expectation because these repairs typically require greater dissection and the creation of a much larger bleeding bone surface compared with smaller tears. However, a review of patients with massive rotator cuff repair reveals a very low incidence of clinically significant postoperative stiffness. This finding is particularly important, as recent studies have shown that massive rotator cuff repairs are at an increased risk for retearing and that methods to reduce strains across the repair during healing should be used.[3] Perhaps part of the explanation for the low incidence of stiffness in these patients is that arthroscopic repair is done with minimal dissection relative to open repair.

There are many benefits of using arthroscopic techniques for treatment of rotator cuff pathology. For one, the limited nature of dissection across tissue planes results in less scar tissue and adhesion formation. This tendency toward less scar formation supports the use of a conservative rehabilitation program after arthroscopic repair of large and massive rotator cuff tears to maximize the opportunity for tendon to bone healing. The same principles apply to smaller tears, as minimizing tissue plane disruptions and scar formation allow surgeons the freedom to delay the initiation of motion that may potentially disrupt the surgical repair.

SUMMARY

A rehabilitation program that best allows for tendon to bone healing while preventing shoulder stiffness is the goal after arthroscopic rotator cuff repairs. A customized rehabilitation program based on risk factors for developing postoperative stiffness helps to achieve these goals.

Experience with rotator cuff surgery has enabled the authors to develop differential rehabilitation guidelines in selected patient categories that are predisposed toward postoperative stiffness (ie, patients with preoperative calcific tendinitis, adhesive capsulitis, labral tear requiring repair, single-tendon supraspinatus tears, and/or PASTA lesions). In these stiffness-prone categories, a modified protocol has successfully been instituted by using more aggressive closed-chain stretching exercises in the early postoperative period for patients with any of the risk factors. The results of this postoperative regimen have been encouraging, and the authors enthusiastically recommend it. Patients who develop refractory postoperative stiffness are effectively treated with arthroscopic capsular release and lysis of adhesions. In these instances, the original pathology is reliably healed by the time of arthroscopic release. Patients regain motion, and they are satisfied after the operation. Patients who do not fall into the high-risk category are treated with the conservative rehabilitation protocol.

REFERENCES

1. Millett PJ, Wilcox RB 3rd, O'Holleran JD, et al. Rehabilitation of the rotator cuff: an evaluation-based approach. J Am Acad Orthop Surg 2006;14(11):599–609.
2. Brislin KJ, Field LD, Savoie FH 3rd. Complications after arthroscopic rotator cuff repair. Arthroscopy 2007;23(2):124–8.
3. Galatz LM, Ball CM, Teefey SA, et al. The outcome and repair integrity of completely arthroscopically repaired large and massive rotator cuff tears. J Bone Joint Surg Am 2004;86-A(2):219–24.
4. Thomazeau H, Boukobza E, Morcet N, et al. Prediction of rotator cuff repair results by magnetic resonance imaging. Clin Orthop Relat Res 1997;(344):275–83.
5. Lo IK, Burkhart SS. Arthroscopic revision of failed rotator cuff repairs: technique and results. Arthroscopy 2004;20(3):250–67.
6. Huberty DP, Schoolfield JD, Brady PC, et al. Incidence and treatment of postoperative stiffness following arthroscopic rotator cuff repair. Arthroscopy 2009;25(8): 880–90.
7. Verma NN, Ferry AT, Bhatia S, et al. Arthroscopic management of stiffness following rotator cuff repair: techniques and results. Arthroscopy 2009;25(6):e2.

8. Bey MJ, Song HK, Wehrli FW, et al. Intratendinous strain fields of the intact supraspinatus tendon: the effect of glenohumeral joint position and tendon region. J Orthop Res 2002;20(4):869–74.
9. Bey MJ, Ramsey ML, Soslowsky LJ. Intratendinous strain fields of the supraspinatus tendon: effect of a surgically created articular-surface rotator cuff tear. J Shoulder Elbow Surg 2002;11(6):562–9.
10. Burkhart SS, Klein JR. Arthroscopic repair of rotator cuff tears associated with large bone cysts of the proximal humerus: compaction bone grafting technique. Arthroscopy 2005;21(9):1149.
11. Sonnabend D. Healing of torn rotator cuff tendon. Presented at the 10th International Congress of Shoulder and Elbow Surgery. Costa do Sauipe, Brazil, September 18, 2007.
12. Warner JJ, Greis PE. The treatment of stiffness of the shoulder after repair of the rotator cuff. Instr Course Lect 1998;47:67–75.
13. Flurin PH, Landreau P, Gregory T, et al. [Arthroscopic repair of full-thickness cuff tears: a multicentric retrospective study of 576 cases with anatomical assessment.]. Rev Chir Orthop Reparatrice Appar Mot 2005;91(S8):31–42 [in French].
14. Severud EL, Ruotolo C, Abbott DD, et al. All-arthroscopic versus mini-open rotator cuff repair: a long-term retrospective outcome comparison. Arthroscopy 2003;19(3):234–8.
15. Tauro JC. Stiffness and rotator cuff tears: incidence, arthroscopic findings, and treatment results. Arthroscopy 2006;22(6):581–6.

Rehabilitation of Acromioclavicular Joint Separations: Operative and Nonoperative Considerations

Mark P. Cote, PT, DPT[a], Karen E. Wojcik, MSPT, ATC[b], Gregg Gomlinski, MSPT, CSCS[b], Augustus D. Mazzocca, MS, MD[a,*]

KEYWORDS

- Acromioclavicular joint • Acromioclavicular separation
- Rehabilitation approach

Acromioclavicular joint (AC) separations are one of the most common injuries seen in orthopedic and sports medicine practices, accounting for 9% of all injuries to the shoulder girdle.[1–3] Various operative and nonoperative treatment schemes have been described for the management of AC joint injuries.[4–33] Although considerable controversy exists over the efficacy of surgical reconstruction versus nonoperative intervention for grade III type injuries, grade I and II separations seem to respond favorably to conservative management. Conversely, grades IV, V, and VI often require surgical reconstruction. Regardless of the type of injury, rehabilitation as a part of conservative management and postoperative care plays an important role in the management of these injuries. This article presents the authors' rehabilitation approach to treatment of acromioclavicular separations pre- and postoperatively.

CONCEPTUAL FRAMEWORK

To provide instruction and insight for rehabilitation clinicians, protocols are often provided for a specific injury or procedure. A protocol is a system of rules or procedures for a given situation. Although intended to be informative, protocols often result in a restrictive list of exercises and arbitrary time frames that a clinician is expected to

[a] Department of Orthopaedic Surgery, University of Connecticut Health Center, Medical Arts & Research Building, Room 4017, 263 Farmington Avenue, Farmington, CT 06034, USA
[b] Department of Rehabilitation Services, University of Connecticut Health Center, Farmington, CT, USA
* Corresponding author.
E-mail address: admazzocca@yahoo.com (A.D. Mazzocca).

Clin Sports Med 29 (2010) 213–228
doi:10.1016/j.csm.2009.12.002
sportsmed.theclinics.com

follow. It is the authors' experience that protocols tend to diminish a clinician's ability to provide quality patient care by discouraging critical thinking and clinical decision making by providing a predetermined set of care plans. Furthermore, protocols assume that each patient arrives at the same rehabilitation milestone at the same point in time.

When discussing the approach to rehabilitation the authors believe it is best to outline guidelines based on anatomy, pathoanatomy, and biologic healing for the progression of activities. Providing the rationale for rehabilitative services enables rehabilitation clinicians to use their entire skill set in a safe and efficient manner, thereby maximizing the quality of care provided to patients. Considering this conceptual approach to rehabilitation, the following rehabilitation guidelines are presented for the management of AC joint separations.

NONOPERATIVE MANAGEMENT

Historically, grade I and II AC separations have been managed nonoperatively with periods of immobilization and rehabilitation.[26–31] Although nonoperative treatment is generally accepted as the treatment of choice for these injuries, evidence to support the efficacy of rehabilitation protocols is limited to case series (level IV) and expert opinion (level V). Mouhsine and colleagues[27] reported on 33 grade I and II AC separations treated conservatively with immobilization and physical therapy. At 6.3 years post treatment, the mean constant score was 82, with 17 of 33 subjects (52%) remaining asymptomatic. Of those patients with residual symptoms, 9 (27%) required surgical intervention to address continued pain and dysfunction.[27] Bergfeld and colleagues[26] examined the results of conservative treatment and the management of grade I and II AC separations in US Naval Academy shipmen. Their results demonstrated 30% of grade I and 42% of grade II separations presented with complaints of pain and clicking with push-ups and dips on follow-up. Furthermore, persistent pain and limitation of activities were present in 9% of type I and 23% of type II injuries.[26]

Literature to support the efficacy of specific rehabilitation protocols is also limited. Gladstone and colleagues[28] described a 4-part physical therapy protocol for the treatment of grade I, II, and III AC joint injuries in athletes. Phase 1 focuses on the elimination of pain and protection of the AC joint through sling immobilization (3–10 days), along with the prevention of muscular atrophy. Phase 2 consists of range of motion exercises to restore full mobility and a gradual progression of strengthening with the addition of isotonic exercise. Phase 3 involves advanced strengthening to enhance the dynamic stability of the AC joint. Phase 4 incorporates sport-specific training to prepare for a full return to prior level of activity.[28]

The guidelines set here follow those outlined by Gladstone and colleagues. The goal of rehabilitation is to return the patient to the previous level of activity. Return to full activity depends on how well the AC joint is able to function, which depends on the ability to maximize dynamic stability of the AC joint through strength training of the supporting muscles of the shoulder girdle and the avoidance of degenerative joint disease associated with these injuries. Advancements in rehabilitation programs are based on the reduction of pain and inflammation, restoration of range of motion, improvements in strength, and ability to perform sport-, work-, or function-specific tasks without limitations. These theoretic concepts form the basis of directing nonoperative care.

GRADE I

A grade I separation involves a sprain of the AC ligaments without clavicle displacement, theoretically resulting in little insult to joint stability.[1] In this instance, the authors do not insist on a sling. If patients in the acute phases of injury are experiencing significant pain and discomfort, a sling may be used to reduce stress on the AC joint to encourage cessation of pain and further inflammation. The criteria for discharge of the sling include the absence of pain with the arm at the side and during self-care activities. Early initiation of range of motion activities assists in reducing pain and inflammation and expedites discharge from the sling. Historically, a Kenny Howard sling has been advocated as an effective means of immobilizing the AC joint. However, problems associated with the device, specifically skin breakdown, have led many clinicians to discontinue its use.[33,34]

Mobility exercises are initiated within the first week of injury in an effort to decrease associated morbidity. Initial goals are to restore mobility by gradually progressing shoulder range of motion with supervised and home exercises and manual therapy techniques, specifically passive range of motion. Ranges of motion that may increase stress on the AC joint, specifically internal rotation (IR) behind the back, cross-body adduction, and end-range forward elevation, are approached cautiously and within a patient's own pain threshold; however, they are not expressly limited as stability is less of a concern than in higher-grade separations. Following a week of rehabilitation, restrictions in passive or active shoulder motion are uncommon. In patients with persistent limitations in shoulder mobility lasting greater than a week, concomitant or separate diagnoses should be considered.

Strength exercise is begun immediately and progressed according to the patient's tolerance to activity. In the authors' experience, accelerating exercises by moving through acutely painful and stressful ranges of motions tends to encourage continued pain and inflammation, making it difficult if not impossible to maintain improvements in mobility or strength. By allowing exercises to be progressed within the guidelines of AC joint pain patients can maximize their own potential for progress.

Closed-chain scapular exercises similar to those described by Burkhart and colleagues[35] and McMullen and Uhl[36] are recommended as an introductory exercise to assist in isolating scapular movements. The term closed-chain refers to exercises in which the distal segment is fixed.[37] In shoulder rehabilitation, closed-chain exercises involve movements with the hand fixed to a wall, table, or floor. These exercises unload the weight of the arm, thereby minimizing the demand of the rotator cuff musculature to support the weight of the arm.[36] These exercises are adventitious as they allow patients to focus on quality, appropriate movements in a safe and pain-free manner. Examples of these exercises include scapular clocks (**Fig. 1**A) and scapular protraction and retraction on the wall (**Fig. 1**B).

The addition of isotonic and open-chain exercises can be made when the patient is able to maintain positions of forward elevation without pain or weakness. Exercise is progressed with isotonic strength exercises, focusing on the scapular and rotator cuff musculature, followed by sport-, work-, or function-specific training (**Fig. 2**). A return to sport or work activity that is dependent on symptom-free demonstration of task-specific activity can occur as early as 2 weeks.

GRADE II

A grade II separation involves tearing of the AC ligaments, potentially resulting in anteroposterior movement of the clavicle.[1] Grade II separations do not involve the coracoclavicular ligaments and thus superior to inferior displacement of the clavicle is less of a concern. Similar to grade I separations, grade II separations are only immobilized acutely to manage pain and inflammation. During this period of immobilization, the authors allow pain to guide sling use. In grade II separations some healing of the AC ligaments may occur. In the early periods of tissue healing, active range of motion

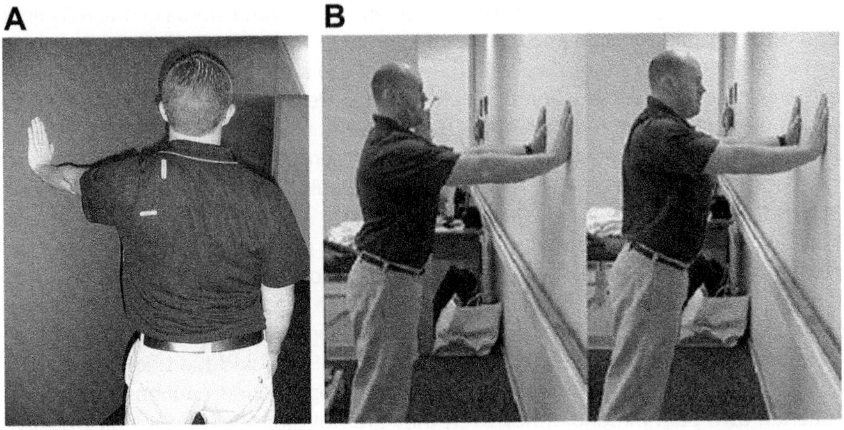

Fig. 1. Closed-chain exercises. Scapular clocks (*A*) scapular protraction/retraction against wall (*B*).

and self-care activities may be accompanied by pain, indicating the need for further protection with continued use of a sling. Following the cessation of pain at rest with the arm at the side and with self-care activities, immobilization is discontinued.

Given the tearing of the AC ligaments and the potential for increases in posterior to anterior movement of the clavicle, the authors suggest immediate initiation of scapular exercises, emphasizing retraction to provide dynamic stability to the AC joint. Several exercises for scapular retraction have been described.[38–42] In the author's experience, rehabilitation clinicians prescribe exercises based on the amount of selective muscle activity they produce. From this perspective, horizontal abduction with external rotation and prone horizontal extension with the arm at 100°[43] (Blackburn exercises, or "Ts" and "Ys") would seem desirable as they have been shown to elicit high levels of muscle activity of the middle and lower trapezius[40] (see **Fig. 2**C). These exercises have also been shown to produce high amounts of electromyographic activity of the supraspinatus and infraspinatus.[44–46] In addition, the positioning of the upper extremity creates a long lever arm, producing high amounts of stress in the AC joint, which makes these exercises less tolerable in the acute and subacute phases of injury.

The authors prefer to start with closed-chain scapular activities that are easily tolerated early in the postinjury period, allowing the patient to work on scapular strength and motion without provoking undesirable increases in symptoms. These exercises unload the weight of the upper extremity, allowing the patient to focus on isolating scapular motion. For example, patients performing a scapular clock positioned with their hand on the wall are instructed to position the scapula in depression or somewhere between 6:00 and 7:30 for a right shoulder and between 6:00 and 4:30 for a left shoulder. This exercise can be treated as an isometric activity by instructing the patient to maintain the position through sustained muscle contraction for 10 seconds or more depending on tolerance to the activity (**Fig. 3**).

Continued attention is paid toward the patient's ability to maintain scapular retraction as symptoms continue to abate. To advance this, rowing exercises with tubing or cable resistance are initiated to integrate combined motions of the upper extremity. Early integration of kinetic chain exercises is also recommended to enhance recovery of shoulder function and improve the patient's ability to produce and maintain scapular retraction. Based on the kinetic link model, these exercises combine leg and trunk

A

B

C

D

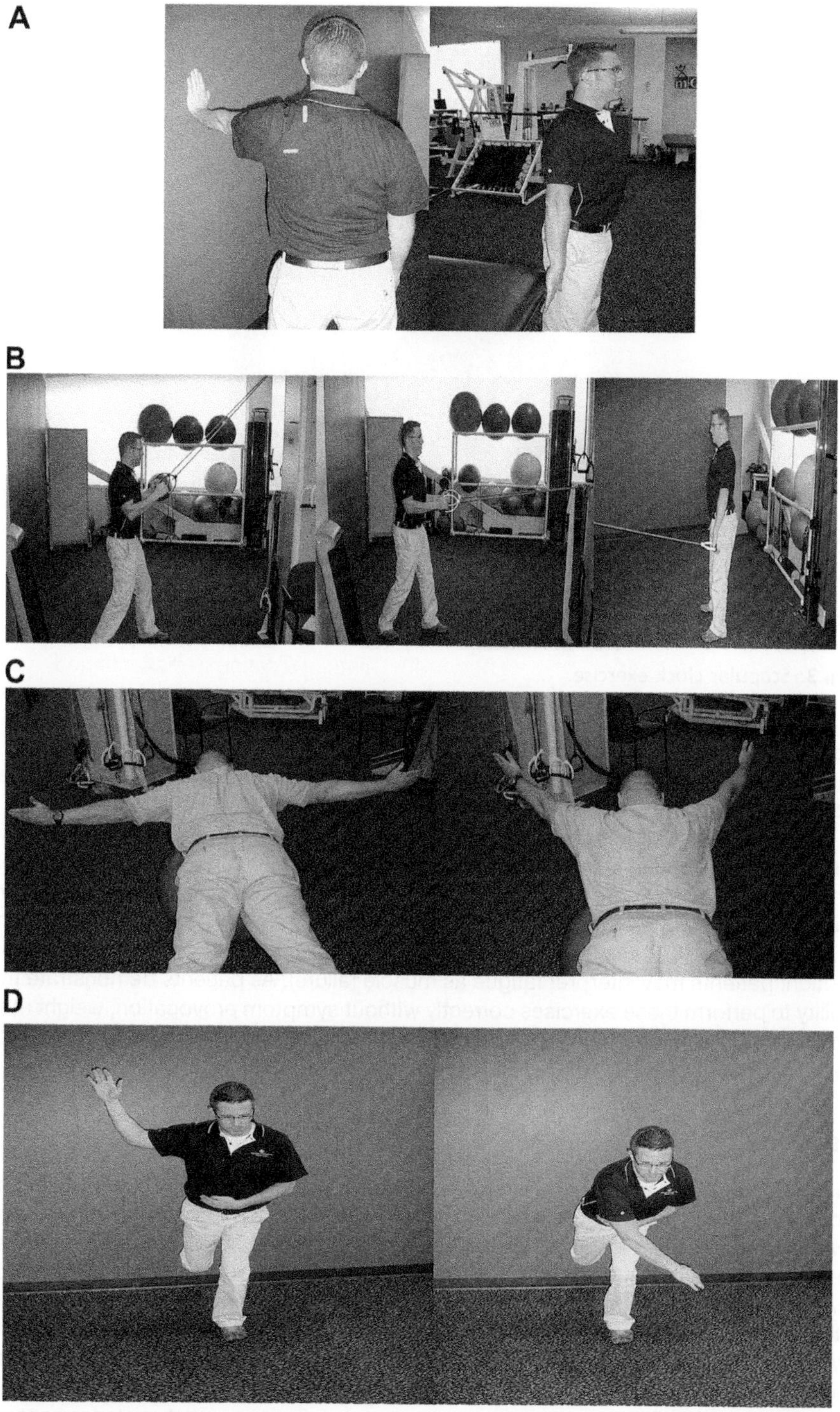

Fig. 2. (*A*) Closed-chain activities: scapular clocks, isometric low row. (*B*) Isotonic 3-level rowing. (*C*) Horizontal abduction with external rotation (physiotherapy ball T [*left*]) and prone horizontal extension with the arm at 100° (physiotherapy ball Y [*right*]). (*D*) Sports-specific exercise: disco exercise that may mimic overhead sport activities.

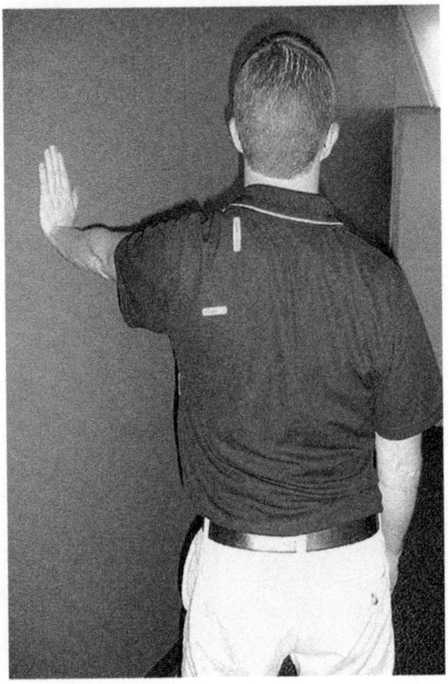

Fig. 3. Scapular clock exercise.

activity with shoulder motions to reinforce normally occurring movement patterns of the upper extremity.[36,47] The lawn-mower and disco motions are examples of commonly prescribed kinetic chain exercises (**Fig. 4**).

As the patient demonstrates increases in strength and the ability to tolerate activities with the arm extended in front of the body, horizontal abduction with external rotation and prone horizontal extension with the arm at 100° can be introduced into the exercise program (see **Fig. 2**C). The authors prefer to start these exercises with no weight with sets performed to fatigue (defined as the inability to correctly perform the exercise motion; patients may interpret fatigue as muscle failure). As patients demonstrate the ability to perform these exercises correctly without symptom provocation, weight may be added. Return to full activity can occur once the patient can demonstrate the ability to perform task-specific activity related to his or her sport or work.

GRADE III

In considering treatment options for patients who have sustained grade III AC separations, consulting the literature reveals a lack of publications supporting one approach over another. This finding is evident in Spencer's[48] systematic review of the literature, in which comprehensive search strategies revealed studies with only low levels of evidence appropriate for data analysis. The results of this review supported nonoperative management over surgical reconstruction based primarily on the lack of definitive data demonstrating improved outcomes with operative treatment. Furthermore, higher complication rates, longer recovery, and increased time away from work and sport associated with operative management were offered as a rationale for conservative rehabilitation versus surgical intervention.[48] A recent systematic review by Ceccarelli and colleagues[49] revealed 640 articles regarding AC dislocation, only 5 of which were appropriate for data analysis. The results of that review led the

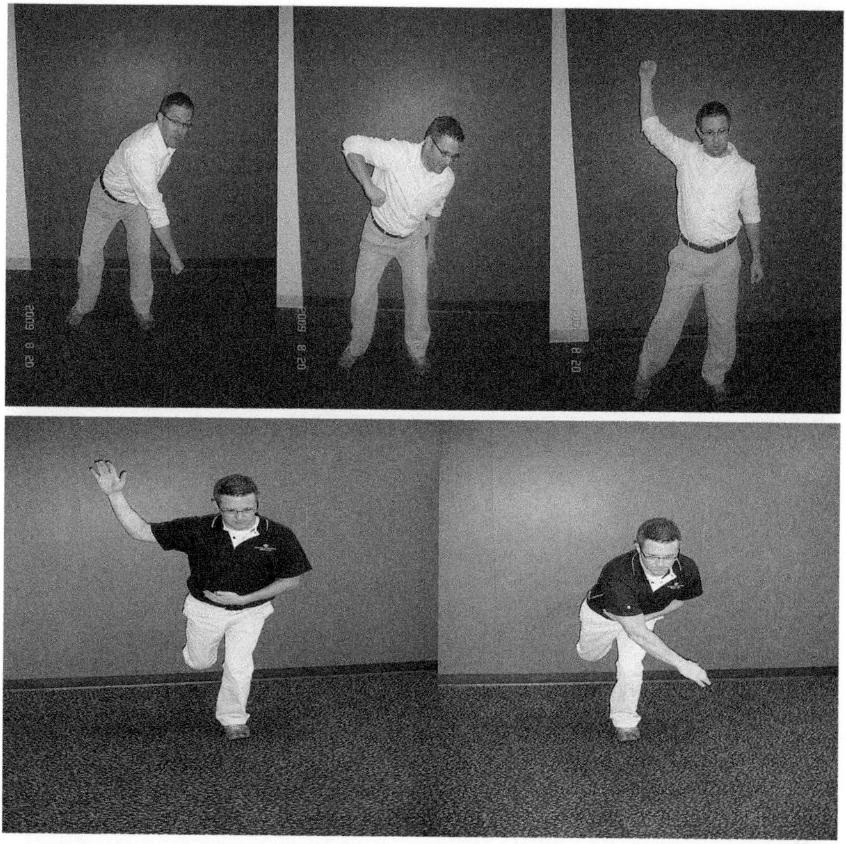

Fig. 4. Double-limb stance initiating lawn mower exercises with an overhead follow-through for work- or sport-specific motions, (*bottom*) advanced to single leg. Note the arm in the bottom image is in a protected position, or a sling can also be used to protect the healing AC joint.

investigators to conclude that although operative and nonoperative management produced comparable results, surgery was associated with higher rates of complications.[49] Nissen and Chatterjee[50] surveyed the American Orthopaedic Society for Sports Medicine (AOSSM) and approved Accreditation Council for Graduate Medical Education (ACGME) orthopedic program residency directors to determine practice preferences in the management of uncomplicated grade III separations; they found that more than 80% opt for conservative management.[50]

Grade III AC separations involve complete disruption of the acromioclavicular and coracoclavicular ligaments, resulting in 100% superior displacement of the clavicle.[1] Complete ligament rupture offers little or no potential for healing and thus immobilization is strictly used to reduce initial pain and inflammation. The authors suggest minimal immobilization and immediate initiation of rehabilitation to decrease pain and inflammation. Although sling use up to 4 weeks following grade III AC separations has been previously reported, patients should be encouraged to cease sling use as soon as their symptoms allow. The AC joint functions primarily through movement of the acromion on the stable strut of the clavicle, producing motion that contributes to total shoulder mobility. In grade III separations the stability of the AC joint is significantly compromised. The loss of the acromioclavicular ligaments allows unopposed anterior to posterior movement of the clavicle, although the loss of integrity of the coracoclavicular ligaments produces superior displacement of the clavicle, which results in significant alterations in the attachment of the scapula to the clavicle. Treatment directed toward scapular stabilization is essential for successful management of grade III AC injuries nonoperatively.

The authors' standard of care is to treat all grade III AC separations with a 6- to 12-week trial of rehabilitation to maximize functional recovery (**Fig 5**). A 6- to 12-week period of rehabilitation is a valuable prognostic indicator for predicting ability to return to sport or work activity. In the authors' experience, patients who go on to need operative intervention typically demonstrate little to no response after 6 weeks

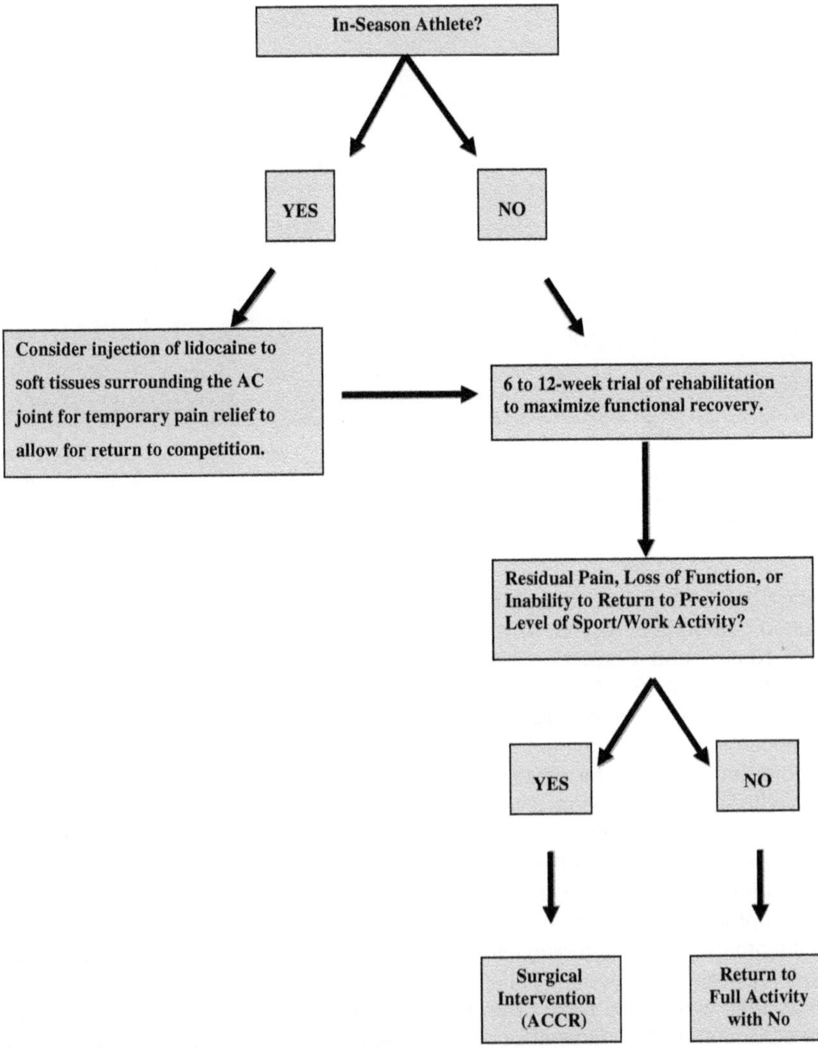

Fig. 5. Algorithmic approach to the management of grade III AC separations.

of rehabilitation. Conversely, those patients who have had a significant reduction in symptoms in the first 6 weeks are allowed to resume sport- or work-specific activities and are encouraged to continue rehabilitation up to 12 weeks. Provided a patient can safely perform required work or sport activity and has no activity-limiting pain, return to full activity is permitted. These patients, although successfully returning to their desired level of activity, require continued follow-up as functional decline may still occur. In these cases, rehabilitation is formally resumed and progressed accordingly. Those patients who are not responsive to rehabilitation either initially or as a result of continued relapse are offered operative intervention with anatomic coracoclavicular reconstruction (ACCR).

Those patients who continue with conservative care follow the same progression as described for grade II AC separations, starting with closed-chain exercises to improve scapular control, moving to combined motions with Thera-Band tubing (Hygenic Corporation, Akron, OH, USA) or cable resistance, and finally open-chain exercises and sport- or work-specific training. This progression is initiated immediately and progressed according to the patient's ability to tolerate exercise without provocation of symptoms. The amount of tissue trauma involved in grade III separations is greater than that associated with grades I and II, typically resulting in increased levels of pain and discomfort. In the acute and subacute phases of injury when these symptoms are typically present, lower extremity and core exercises focusing on kinetic chain strength and control are recommended as these exercises play a role in achieving scapular stabilization and can be performed with minimal or no use of the arm. These exercises can be later modified to incorporate the use of the shoulder as the patient's ability to tolerate upper extremity activities improve. As symptoms continue to subside and the ability to perform scapular exercise improves, advanced scapular exercises, such as Blackburn Ts and Ys can be initiated to maximize scapular strength.

Achieving and maintaining scapular control is imperative for successful nonoperative management. On physical examination, patients with grade III AC separations often present with alterations in scapula position and movement. Gumina and colleagues[51] evaluated scapular abnormalities in patients with chronic grade III AC separations. Scapular positioning statically and dynamically was assessed according to the Kibler rating system (scapular dyskinesis) and the Morgan grading scheme (SICK scapula [scapular malposition, inferior medial scapular winging, coracoid tenderness, and scapular dyskinesis]). Scapular dyskinesis was present in 70.6% of patients, of whom 58.3% had SICK scapula syndrome. Those patients with existing scapular dykinesis demonstrated lower constant and simple shoulder scores. Similarly, in the authors' experience patients with persistent scapular abnormalities typically present with low outcome scores, having not responded to nonoperative rehabilitation.[51]

Several bracing options for facilitating and scapular retraction have been advocated. A clavicle or figure-of-eight brace has been used to retract the scapula manually. This brace can be useful for assisting in controlling excessive scapular protraction; however, assistance is typically required to don and doff it, often leading to poor tolerance. Newer options include the S3 brace, a shirtlike compression device that is secured with adjustable neoprene and Velcro straps designed in part to promote optimal scapular positioning. The S3 system can be a useful addition to a rehabilitation program, assisting patients in maintaining a retracted position of the scapula. Strapless posture apparel is also ideal for encouraging scapular retraction. IntelliSkin "proprioposture support" shirts use the same concepts as the S3 brace to promote posture and optimal scapular positioning.

GRADES IV, V, VI

Grade IV, V, and VI AC separations are treated operatively with ACCR. The authors have had some incidental success with nonoperative management of grade V separations. Some patients who opt out of surgical reconstruction have followed the nonoperative guidelines with some success. There may be several reasons for this. First, these patients tend to be more than 55 years of age and are generally involved in activities that place low demand on the shoulder. Second, there may be some selection bias as these patients were resistant to operative intervention and self-selected a course of nonoperative management. The diagnostic criteria to distinguish between a grade III and grade V separation may inadvertently lead to a false-negative result. A grade V separation results in 300% displacement of the clavicle, whereas a grade III accounts for 100%.[1] In cases in which a clavicular displacement exceeds 100% the diagnosis of grade V may be made regardless of whether the displacement meets the 300% that defines a true grade V.

POSTOPERATIVE REHABILITATION FOLLOWING ACCR

Patients with persistent symptoms and functional limitations recalcitrant to nonoperative rehabilitation are offered surgical intervention. Several operative procedures have been described for restoring stability to the AC joint, all of which require some form of biologic healing. Postoperative rehabilitation needs to be tailored according to tissue-healing time frames.

The senior author's preferred method of reconstruction is ACCR. The goal of this procedure is to restore the anatomy and return stability to the AC joint. This goal is accomplished by reconstructing the coracoclavicular ligaments with a soft-tissue allograft that is passed around the underside of the coracoid and up through 2 bone tunnels that have been drilled in the clavicle at the approximate insertion site of the native ligaments. Fixation is achieved using 2 interference anchors, 1 in each bone tunnel. By restoring the anatomy of the coracoclavicular ligaments the body is able to undergo the biologic healing process it was previously unable to achieve when the ligaments were completely torn. As patients enter the postoperative period, they are also just beginning the healing process.

The authors' guidelines for progression of activities following ACCR are based on the tissue-healing time frames on tendon healing in a bone tunnel. Rodeo and colleagues[52] examined healing response following the placement of a tendon graft in a bone tunnel in a canine model, and found construct failure through pull-out of the tendon from the tunnel on load-to-failure testing at 2, 4, and 8 weeks. At 12 weeks or more, failure occurred at the midsubstance of the tendon, indicating adequate healing at the bone-tendon interface.[52] Subsequent research has shown similar findings for tendon healing in a bone tunnel.[53]

Considering this research, guidelines have been developed for the progression of activities following ACCR. Preoperatively, patients are counseled in brace use and are taught a postoperative home program involving hand, wrist, and elbow exercise. Postoperatively patients are immobilized in a platform brace (Lerman Shoulder Orthosis, DonJoy Inc, Vista, CA, USA) for 6 to 8 weeks (**Fig. 6**). This brace allows for adequate unloading of the arm, thereby decreasing the amount of stress placed on the surgically reconstructed AC joint. This is an important facet of early postoperative management as the articulation between the clavicle and the acromion is the only link joining the upper extremity to the thorax. Patients are instructed to remain in the brace at all times other than during self-care and prescribed therapeutic activities. Following removal of the brace, patients are referred to rehabilitation for active

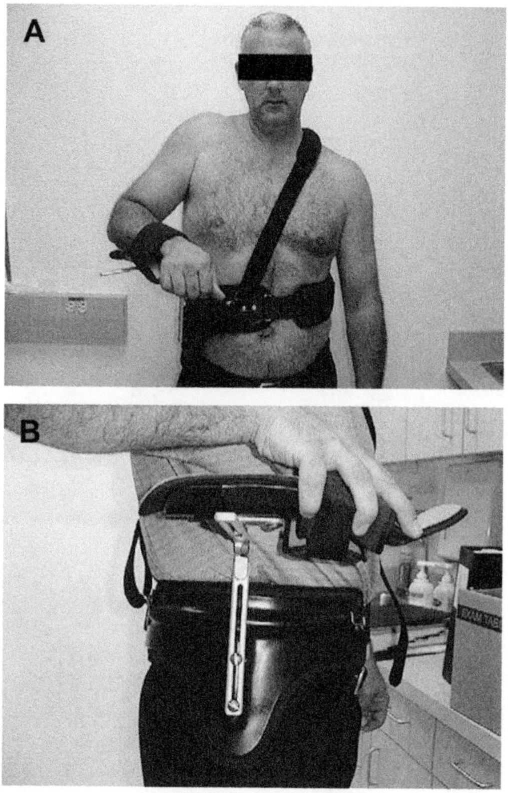

Fig. 6. Lerman brace (*A, B*).

assistive range of motion in all planes. The primary rationale for rehabilitation services is to manage the effects of 6 to 8 weeks of immobilization. Patients coming out of the brace tend to be stiff; however, because of the positioning of the Lerman device, which places the shoulder in external rotation, restrictions in mobility are not typically pronounced.

Similar to nonoperative management, motions that may increase stress on the AC joint, specifically IR behind the back, cross-body adduction, and end-range forward elevation, are approached cautiously and within a patient's own pain threshold. The authors prefer to initiate range of motion exercises with limb-supported activities like the table or wall slide. These closed-chain exercises have been shown to elicit low amounts of shoulder-muscle activity.[54] These exercises can be started on a flat surface and gradually progressed to inclined surfaces and finally a vertical surface. The addition of supine flexion and pulley exercises also assists in increasing forward elevation (**Fig. 7**). The authors' experience indicates patients respond favorably to this progression, as it allows the patient to increase the amount of muscle contribution gradually with each exercise.

In the authors' experience with ACCR procedure, mobility restrictions recalcitrant to rehabilitation have not been observed. At 10 weeks postoperatively, patients typically present with near full restoration of range of motion, lacking only the ability to perform IR behind the back. Stretching exercises behind the back like towel IR are allowed only if the patient can maintain scapular retraction while performing the exercise (**Fig. 8**).

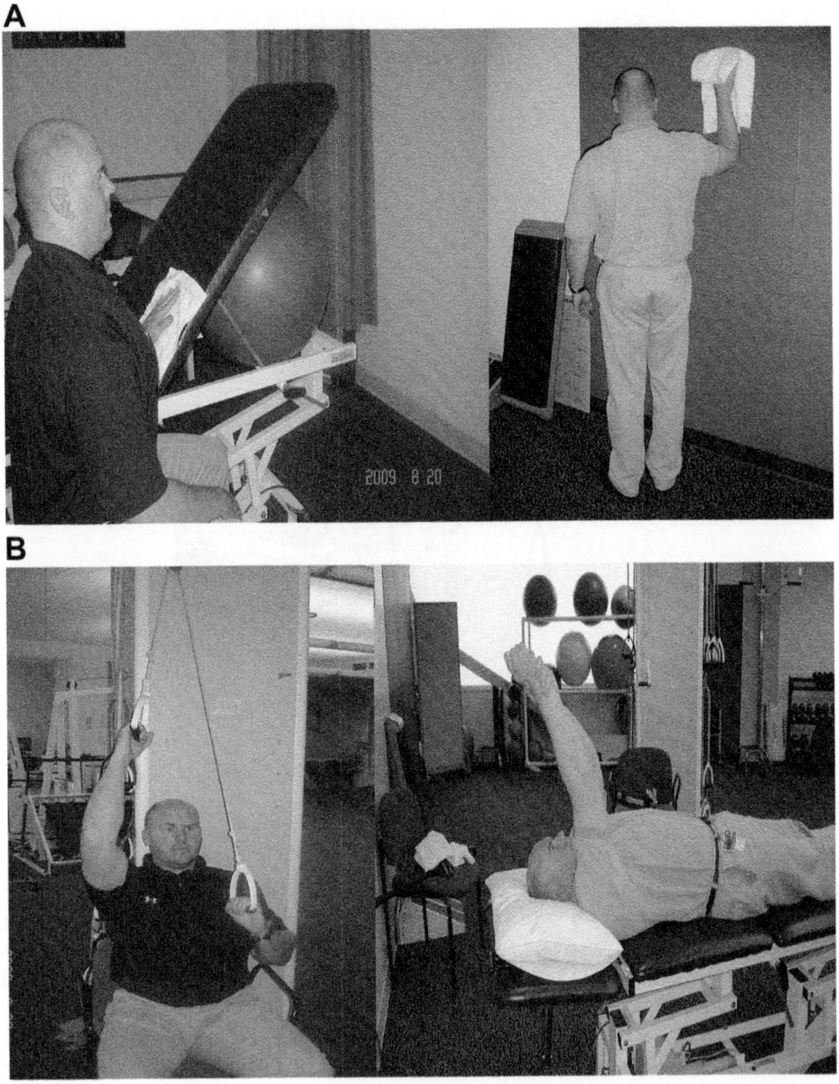

Fig. 7. (*A*) A graduated table slide followed by a wall slide performed in the plane of the scapula. (*B*) Assisted forward elevation with a pulley and supine flexion.

This limitation in motion seems to be related to the mechanics of the AC joint rather than restrictions in glenohumeral joint mobility. Conventional capsular stretching of the glenohumeral joint is typically not needed.

All isotonic strength activities are withheld for 12 weeks because of concern about the ability of the surgical construct to tolerate a repetitively applied load. Closed-chain scapular exercises and kinetic chain activities are allowed starting at 8 weeks. These exercises are adventitious as they allow the patient to focus on scapular control and established movement patterns without creating excessive loads about the AC joint. They have also been shown to be effective in producing muscle activity in the scapular muscles in the early phases of shoulder rehabilitation.[55]

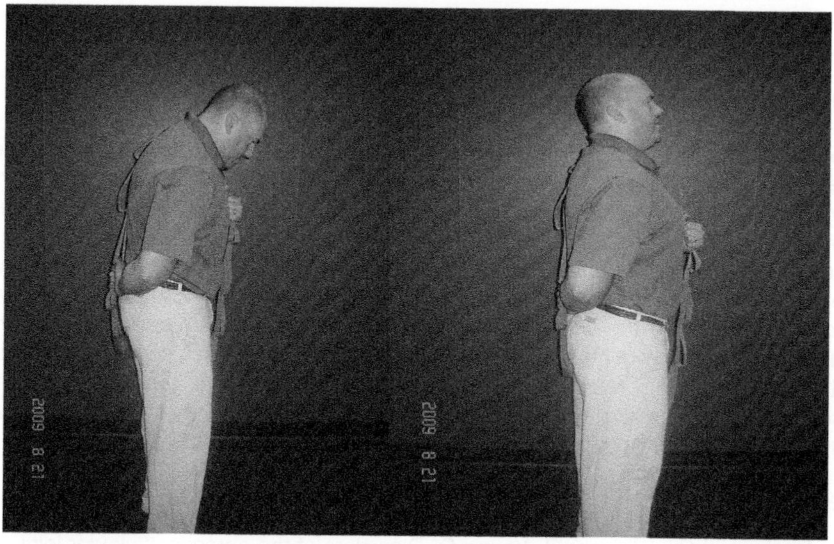

Fig. 8. Towel IR. (*Left*) Poor performance of the IR towel stretch and (*right*) good form (retracted scapula) during IR towel stretch.

From 12 to 18 weeks, exercise is progressed to include isotonic strength activities. The low row is an example of an exercise that transfers well from an isometric to an isotonic strength activity (**Fig. 9**). Multilevel rowing exercises focusing on combined motions with Thera-Band tubing or cable resistance are recommended (see **Fig. 2**B), in addition to continued integration of the legs and trunk, which improves function of the shoulder within the kinetic chain. Advanced strengthening such as

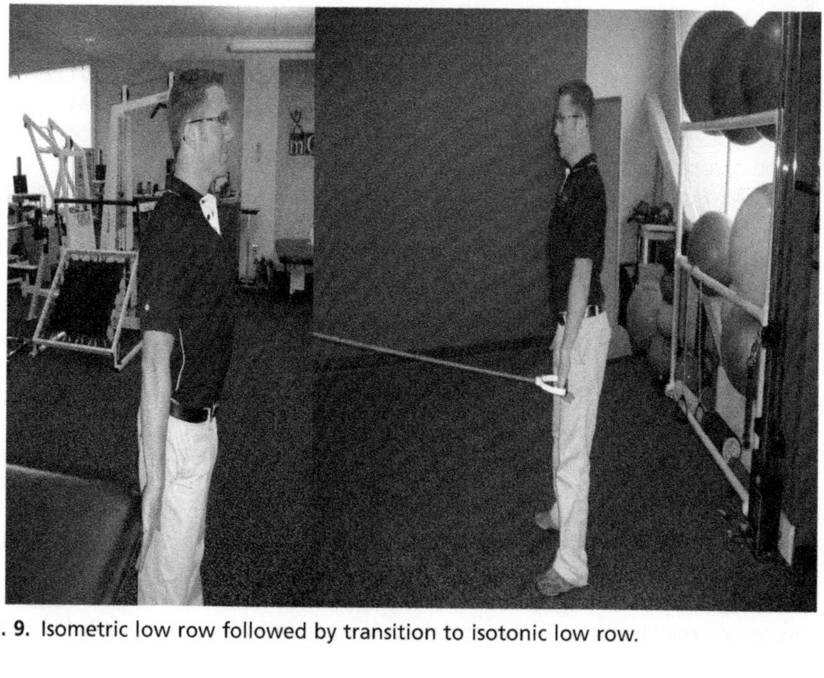

Fig. 9. Isometric low row followed by transition to isotonic low row.

Blackburn exercises can be integrated only after significant scapular control has been demonstrated.

SUMMARY

Regardless of the grade of injury, rehabilitation plays an important role in the management of AC separations. Guidelines based on the anatomy, pathoanatomy, and potential for biologic healing enable rehabilitation clinicians to direct their services appropriately, resulting in optimal patient care. In nonoperative management the sequencing of exercise prescription should match the patient's ability to correctly perform and tolerate rehabilitation activities. Postoperatively, the biologic healing process involved in the surgical procedure needs to be considered with the time frames associated with healing to determine the appropriateness of various rehabilitation activities. With respect to the healing process, exercise can be progressed according to the same principles that guide nonoperative management to maximize patients' recovery from a significant AC joint injury.

REFERENCES

1. Rockwood CJ, Williams G, Young D. Disorders of the acromioclavicular joint. In: Rockwood CJ, Matsen FA III, editors. The shoulder. 2nd edition. Philadelphia: WB Saunders; 1998. p. 483–553.
2. Mazzocca AD, Arciero RA, Bicos J. Evaluation and treatment of acromioclavicular joint injuries. Am J Sports Med 2007;35(2):316–29.
3. Trainer G, Arciero RA, Mazzocca AD. Practical management of grade III acromioclavicular separations. Clin J Sport Med 2008;18(2):162–6.
4. Bosworth BM. Acromioclavicular separation: new method of repair. Surg Gynecol Obstet 1941;73:866–71.
5. Sage FP, Salvatore JE. Injuries of the acromioclavicular joint: a study of results in 96 patients. South Med J 1963;56:486–95.
6. Horn JS. The traumatic anatomy and treatment of acute acromioclavicular dislocation. J Bone Joint Surg Br 1954;36(2):194–201.
7. Weaver JK, Dunn HK. Treatment of acromioclavicular injuries, especially complete acromioclavicular separation. J Bone Joint Surg Am 1972;54(6):1187–94.
8. Mazzocca AD, Conway JE, Johnson SJ, et al. The anatomic coracoclavicular reconstruction. Oper Tech Sports Med 2004;12(1):56–61.
9. Wolf EM, Pennington WT. Arthroscopic reconstruction for acromioclavicular joint dislocation. Arthroscopy 2001;17(5):558–63.
10. Wang S, Du D, Zhang P, et al. A modified method of coracoid transposition for the treatment of complete dislocation of acromioclavicular joint. Chin J Traumatol 2002;5(5):307–10.
11. Rokito AS, Oh YH, Zuckerman JD. Modified Weaver-Dunn procedure or acromioclavicular joint dislocations. Orthopedics 2004;27(1):21–8.
12. Rolla PR, Surace MF, Murena L. Arthroscopic treatment of acute acromioclavicular joint dislocation. Arthroscopy 2004;20(6):662–8.
13. Grutter PW, Petersen SA. Anatomical acromioclavicular ligament reconstruction: a biomechanical comparison of reconstructive techniques of the acromioclavicular joint. Am J Sports Med 2005;33(11):1723–8.
14. Clavert P, Moulinoux P, Kempf J-F. Technique of stabilization in acromioclavicular joint dislocation. Tech Shoulder Elbow Surg 2005;6(1):1–7.
15. Dimakopoulos P, Panagopoulos A, Syggelos SA, et al. Double-loop repair for acute acromioclavicular joint disruption. Am J Sports Med 2006;34(7):1112–9.

16. Chernchujit B, Tischer T, Imhoff AB. Arthroscopic reconstruction of the acromioclavicular joint disruption: surgical technique and preliminary results. Arch Orthop Trauma Surg 2006;126(9):575–81.
17. Struhl S. Double endobutton technique for repair of complete acromioclavicular joint dislocations. Tech Shoulder Elbow Surg 2007;8(4):175–9.
18. Jiang C, Wang M, Rong G. Proximally based conjoined tendon transfer for coracoclavicular reconstruction in the treatment of acromioclavicular dislocation. J Bone Joint Surg Am 2007;89(11):2408–12.
19. Scheibel M, Ifesanya A, Pauly S, et al. Arthroscopically assisted coracoclavicular ligament reconstruction for chronic acromioclavicular joint instability. Arch Orthop Trauma Surg 2008;128(11):1327–33.
20. Wellmann M, Zantop T, Petersen W. Minimally invasive coracoclavicular ligament augmentation with a flip button/polydioxanone repair for treatment of total acromioclavicular joint dislocation. Arthroscopy 2007;23(10):1132.
21. Somers JF, Van der Linden D. Arthroscopic fixation of type III acromioclavicular dislocations. Acta Orthop Belg 2007;73(5):566–70.
22. Lim YW, Sood A, van Riet RP, et al. Acromioclavicular joint reduction, repair and reconstruction using metallic buttons—early results and complications. Tech Shoulder Elbow Surg 2007;8(4):213–21.
23. Tomlinson DP, Altchek DW, Davila J, et al. A modified technique of arthroscopically assisted AC joint reconstruction and preliminary results. Clin Orthop Relat Res 2008;466(3):639–45.
24. Schlegel TF, Burks RT, Marcus RL, et al. A prospective evaluation of untreated acute grade III acromioclavicular separations. Am J Sports Med 2001;29: 699–703.
25. Bradley JP, Elkousy H. Decision making: operative versus nonoperative treatment of acromioclavicular joint injuries. Clin Sports Med 2003;22:277–90.
26. Bergfeld JA, Andrish JT, Clancy WG. Evaluation of the acromioclavicular joint following first- and second-degree sprains. Am J Sports Med 1978;6(4):153–9.
27. Mouhsine E, Garofalo R, Crevoisier X, et al. Grade I and II acromioclavicular dislocations: results of conservative treatment. J Shoulder Elbow Surg 2003;12: 599–602.
28. Gladstone J, Wilk K, Andrews J. Nonoperative treatment of acromioclavicular joint injuries. Oper Tech Sports Med 1997;5:78–87.
29. Galpin RD, Hawkins RJ, Grainger RW. A comparative analysis of operative versus nonoperative treatment of grade III acromioclavicular separations. Clin Orthop Relat Res 1985;193:150–5.
30. Glick JM, Milburn LJ, Haggerty JF, et al. Dislocated acromioclavicular joint: follow-up study of 35 unreduced acromioclavicular dislocations. Am J Sports Med 1977;5:264–70.
31. Rawes ML, Dias JJ. Long-term results of conservative treatment for acromioclavicular dislocation. J Bone Joint Surg Br 1996;78:410–2.
32. Wojtys EM, Nelson G. Conservative treatment of Grade III acromioclavicular dislocations. Clin Orthop Relat Res 1991;(268):112.
33. Allman FL Jr. Fractures and ligamentous injuries of the clavicle and its articulation. J Bone Joint Surg Am 1967;49(4):774–84.
34. Buss DD, Watts JD. Acromioclavicular injuries in the throwing athlete. Clin Sports Med 2003;22(2):327–41, vii.
35. Burkhart SS, Morgan CD, Kibler WB. The disabled throwing shoulder: spectrum of pathology Part III: the SICK scapula, scapular dyskinesis, the kinetic chain, and rehabilitation. Arthroscopy 2003;19(6):641–61.

36. McMullen J, Uhl TL. A kinetic chain approach for shoulder rehabilitation. J Athl Train 2000;35:329–37.
37. Steindler A. Kinesiology of the human body. Springfield (MA): Charles C. Thomas; 1955.
38. Cools AM, Dewitte V, Lanszweert F, et al. Rehabilitation of scapular muscle balance: which exercises to prescribe? Am J Sports Med 2007;35:1744–51.
39. Decker M, Hintermeister R, Faber K, et al. Serratus anterior muscle activity during selected rehabilitation exercises. Am J Sports Med 1999;27:784–91.
40. Ekstrom RA, Donatelli RA, Soderberg GL. Surface electromyographic analysis of exercises for the trapezius and serratus anterior muscles. J Orthrop Sports Phys Ther 2003;33:247–58.
41. Hardwick DH, Beebe JA, McDonnell MK, et al. A comparison of serratus anterior muscle activation during a wall slide exercise and other traditional exercises. J Orthop Sports Phys Ther 2006;36:903–10.
42. Ludewig PM, Hoff MS, Osowski EE, et al. Relative balance of serratus anterior and upper trapezius muscle activity during push-up exercises. Am J Sports Med 2004;32:484–93.
43. Blackburn TA, McLeod WD, White B, et al. EMG analysis of posterior rotator cuff exercises. Athletic Train 1990;25:40–5.
44. Reinold MM, Macrina LC, Wilk KE, et al. Electromyographic analysis of the supraspinatus and deltoid muscles during 3 common rehabilitation exercises. J Athl Train 2007;42:464–9.
45. Reinold MM, Wilk KE, Fleisig GS, et al. Electromyographic analysis of the rotator cuff and deltoid musculature during common shoulder external rotation exercises. J Orthop Sports Phys Ther 2004;34:385–94.
46. Worrell TW, Corey BJ, York SL, et al. An analysis of supraspinatus EMG activity and shoulder isometric force development. Med Sci Sports Exerc 1992;24:744–8.
47. Kibler WB, Livingston BP. Closed chain rehabilitation for the upper and lower extremity. J Am Acad Orthop Surg 2001;9:412–21.
48. Spencer EE Jr. Treatment of grade III acromioclavicular joint injuries: a systematic review. Clin Orthop Relat Res 2007;455:38–44.
49. Ceccarelli E, Bondì R, Alviti F, et al. Treatment of acute grade III acromioclavicular dislocation: a lack of evidence. J Orthop Traumatol 2008;9(2):105–8.
50. Nissen CW, Chatterjee A. Type III acromioclavicular separation: results of a recent survey on its management. Am J Orthop 2007;36(2):89–93.
51. Gumina S, Carbone S, Postacchini F. Scapular dyskinesis and SICK scapula syndrome in patients with chronic type III acromioclavicular dislocation. Arthroscopy 2009;25(1):40–5.
52. Rodeo SA, Arnoczky SP, Torzilli PA, et al. Tendon-healing in a bone tunnel. A biomechanical and histological study in the dog. J Bone Joint Surg Am 1993;75(12):1795–803.
53. St Pierre P, Olson EJ, Elliott JJ, et al. Tendon-healing to cortical bone compared with healing to a cancellous trough. A biomechanical and histological evaluation in goats. J Bone Joint Surg Am 1995;77(12):1858–66.
54. Wise MB, Uhl TL, Mattacola CG, et al. The effect of limb support on muscle activation during shoulder exercises. J Shoulder Elbow Surg 2004;13(6):614–20.
55. Kibler WB, Sciascia AD, Uhl TL, et al. Electromyographic analysis of specific exercises for scapular control in early phases of shoulder rehabilitation. Am J Sports Med 2008;36(9):1789–98.

Rehabilitation of Biceps Tendon Disorders in Athletes

Jessica H.J. Ryu[a], Robert A. Pedowitz, MD, PhD[b,*]

KEYWORDS

- Biceps tendon • Rehabilitation • Shoulder
- Arthroscopy • Tenodesis

The diagnosis and management of an active patient with biceps disease can be challenging for the treating physician. Biceps pathology tends to occur with advancing age and associated rotator cuff injury. A careful review of the function, anatomy, and pathology of biceps in conjunction with a thorough, knowledgeable history and physical examination can yield a working diagnosis in this challenging patient population. Appropriate treatment can be rendered based on the established pathology, be it conservative or surgical. This article focuses on nonsurgical rehabilitation and postoperative rehabilitation of biceps tendon injuries.

KEY POINTS

Anatomy

The origin of the long head of the biceps tendon is derived principally from the posterior labrum with known anatomic variants.[1] In comparison with the distal tendon, the proximal tendon is wider and innervated to a greater extent, with sensory fibers containing substance P and calcitonin gene–related peptide, both of which play a role in vasodilation, plasma extravasation, and pain transmission.[2]

Encased in a synovial sheath, the proximal tendinous portion is 9 cm long and passes through the rotator interval stabilized by a sling composed of the coracohumeral ligament, superior glenohumeral ligament, and fibers from the supraspinatus and subscapularis tendons (**Fig. 1**).[3,4] Once the biceps tendon passes into the bicipital groove, it is covered by the transverse humeral ligament, which we now understand is not the major stabilizing structure of the biceps.[5]

[a] Tulane Medical School, 3915 St Charles Avenue, #209, New Orleans, LA 70115, USA
[b] UCLA/Orthopaedic Hospital—Department of Orthopedic Surgery, David Geffen School of Medicine at UCLA, 10833 Le Conte Avenue, 76-143 CHS, Los Angeles, CA 90095, USA
* Corresponding author.
E-mail address: rpedowitz@mednet.ucla.edu (R.A. Pedowitz).

Clin Sports Med 29 (2010) 229–246
doi:10.1016/j.csm.2009.12.003 sportsmed.theclinics.com

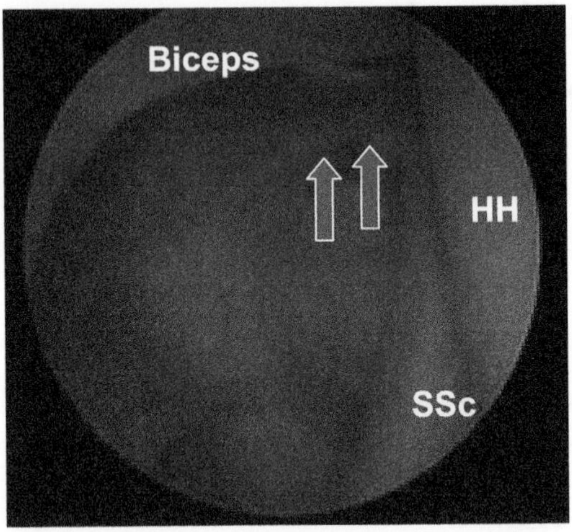

Fig. 1. Medial biceps sling (*arrows*) composed of the coracohumeral ligament, superior glenohumeral ligament, and fibers from the supraspinatus and subscapularis tendons.

Function

The biceps spans from the scapula to the forearm and provides function for the shoulder and the elbow, contributing to elbow flexion and forearm supination. However, the function of biceps specific to the glenohumeral joint is not well understood. Electromyogram data do not consistently support the role of the biceps as a humeral head depressor.[6,7] Some studies suggest that the biceps tendon influences glenohumeral stability,[8] although this contribution is probably a function of the shoulder and elbow position.

Although postulated, the proprioceptive function of the biceps has not been established.[9] Both of the human proximal long bones have muscles that span the 2 adjacent joints on both their dorsal and ventral surfaces (for the humerus, biceps, and triceps and for the femur, quadriceps, and hamstrings). Theoretically, this architecture is well suited to facilitate coordinated proprioceptive feedback and neuromuscular control for the shoulder-elbow and hip-knee combinations, as opposed to maximizing joint torque. However, this theoretical concept is unproven for the biceps tendon specifically.

History and Physical Examination

Patients with shoulder pathology usually present with complaints of pain, weakness, and limited function. These symptoms can result from the stimulation of pain receptors and from tissue failure caused by either microtrauma or macrotrauma. It is critical to establish a functional diagnosis, which permits the treatment of causation rather than simply addressing the symptoms. The physical examination must be thorough and knowledgeable and can be supplemented with tools such as magnetic resonance imaging, computed tomography, high-resolution dynamic ultrasound, and bone scanning.

A detailed and accurate clinical history is essential for establishing a working diagnosis. The history should include questions regarding the onset and duration of symptoms; presence or absence of trauma; provocative factors; and complaints of instability, weakness, clicking, popping, numbness, and tingling.

There are a multitude of physical findings that have been described for the detection of biceps pathology. To date, there is not even one reliable test that can be performed that unequivocally signifies actual biceps pathology. However, there are tests, when positive, that indicate the potential presence of a biceps problem. It is important to palpate the bicipital groove to see if pain is elicited (in comparison with the other shoulder, because this region can normally be a bit sensitive). This is the most useful examination to ascertain possible biceps tendon involvement.[10] Other provocative tests are the Yergason and Speed tests. The Yergason test is performed with the forearm pronated and the elbow flexed to 90°. The physician holds the patient's wrist and provides the resistance against which the patient supinates (**Fig. 2**).[11] For the Speed test, the elbow is extended and the forearm supinated. From this position, the patient elevates his or her hand to 60° against resistance (**Fig. 3**). For both tests, pain in the bicipital groove region may indicate biceps tendon pathology.

Diagnostic Imaging

Although plain radiographs should always be obtained, in most cases the images are normal. The proximal growth plate, the possible presence of an os acromiale, and subacromial stenosis can occur, although on an infrequent basis. The imaging test of choice for the delineation of biceps disease is magnetic resonance imaging and in many centers, a magnetic resonance arthrogram. Important findings include insinuation of contrast material under the biceps anchor or within its substance, implicating a superior labral anterior-to-posterior (SLAP) lesion variant or a partial biceps tear. The biceps as it sits within the bicipital groove is easily visualized, and subluxation or dislocation of the biceps is readily detected on axial images (**Fig. 4**). Failure of contrast material to flow into the bicipital groove may indicate synovitis and stenosis from tendon thickening. Tendonosis and chronic inflammatory changes, best seen on the T2-weighted image, are easily detected in the proximal biceps tendon.

Prevention of biceps injuries in an active individual or an overhead worker should mirror the program undertaken by athletes to limit overuse injuries.[4] Proper stretching, selective strengthening, and ergonomic considerations can help minimize biceps and rotator cuff pathology.[4]

Nonsurgical Rehabilitation

With most biceps pathology, a careful examination will yield an injury amenable to conservative treatment. In general, the first steps in the nonoperative regimen include rest, ice, antiinflammatory medication, and activity modification.[12] Physical therapy

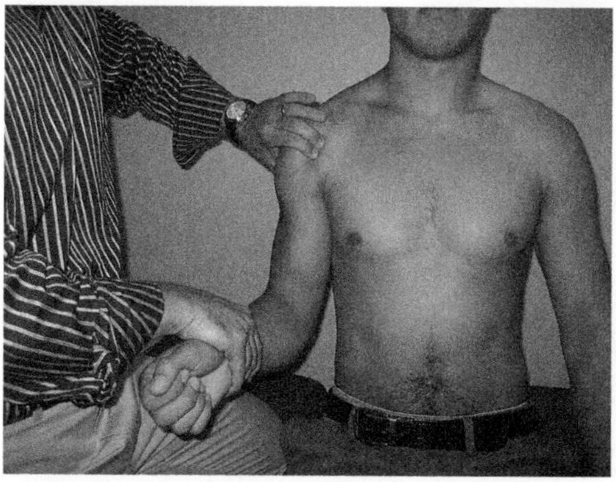

Fig. 2. Yergason test. Forearm flexed to 90° with supination against resistance, eliciting pain in the anterior shoulder.

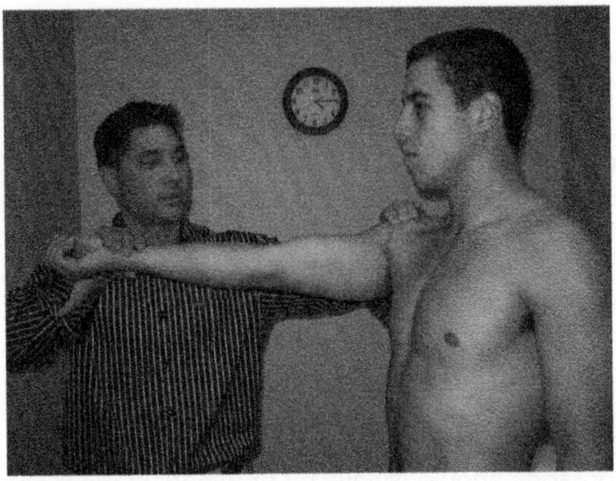

Fig. 3. Speed test. Arm extended and supinated with resisted forward elevation, eliciting pain in anterior shoulder.

can also be an option, depending on the patient's level of pain, with a focus on establishing a pain-free full range of motion, trunk and core stabilization (**Figs. 5** and **6**), and proper scapulothoracic mechanics (**Figs. 7** and **8**), followed by rotator cuff and biceps functional strengthening.

Occasionally, for recalcitrant cases, corticosteroid injections are used. Depending on the presenting pathology, including whether or not the rotator cuff is involved, the physician can give an injection into the subacromial space or the biceps tendon sheath itself (if the major pathology is felt to be isolated to the bicipital groove).[12] An intra-articular injection can also be helpful in those patients with proximal biceps tendon involvement.[5]

There is a paucity of published literature pertaining to the nonoperative treatment of isolated biceps tendon pathology. A Cochrane systematic review analyzing 26 trials of physical therapy for shoulder conditions determined that there was some evidence to support mobilization and exercise in rotator cuff disease; however, the long head of the biceps was not specifically addressed.[13] This most likely reflects the close association between biceps and rotator cuff disease while emphasizing the uncommon

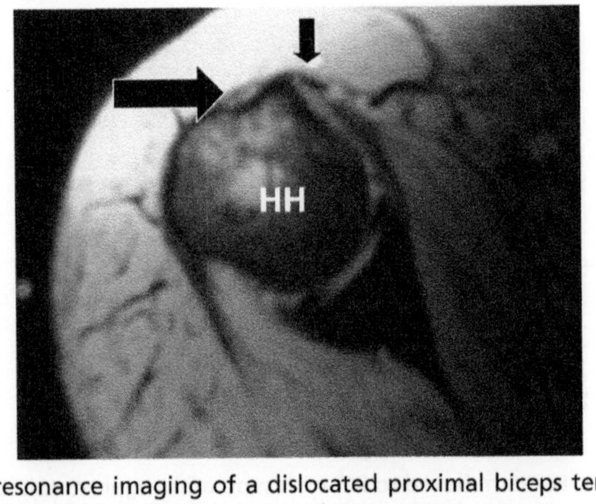

Fig. 4. Magnetic resonance imaging of a dislocated proximal biceps tendon. Small arrow indicates the dislocated biceps. Large arrow points to empty groove.

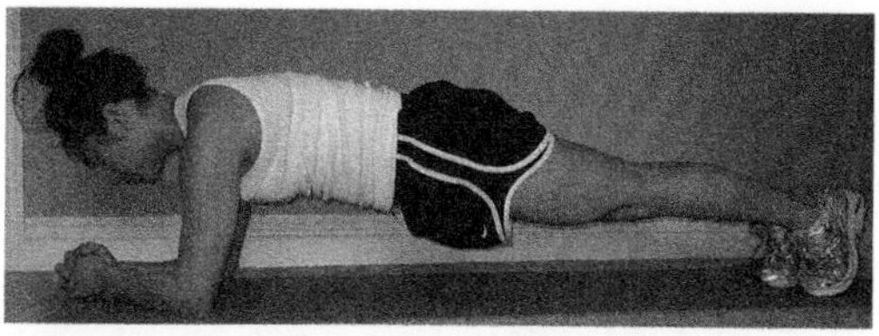

Fig. 5. Forearm plank designed to strengthen core muscles.

occurrence of isolated biceps pathology. Physical therapy, per se, is not the key objective for nonoperative rehabilitation. Rather, our goal should be to work with the patient to develop a proper combination of individualized rehabilitation strategies that they can use and carry forward beyond the phase of hands-on physical therapy.

Based on current recommendations, the following section outlines conservative treatment options for different biceps tendon pathologies.

Primary Biceps Tendonitis

Biceps tendonitis can occur as either primary or secondary inflammation, with the process greatly influenced by the duration of the condition and the patient age.[14] Primary tendonitis, usually resulting from overuse, is an isolated inflammation within the bicipital groove without associated shoulder pathology.[12] Inflammation of the biceps tendon sheath (tenosynovitis) is thought to account for only 5% of tendonitis cases.[15] A review by Ruotolo and colleagues[16] includes a study in which Gross described tenosynovitis within the bicipital groove and noted that this pathology may occur in isolation or in conjunction with rotator cuff disease (**Fig. 9**). Initial treatment of tenosynovitis consisted of nonoperative measures, but for those who failed, the transverse humeral ligament was released arthroscopically to relieve pressure on the confined tendon.

For primary biceps tendonitis, conservative treatment is the initial choice.[17] Rest, ice, and nonsteroidal medications are included in this first line of treatment. Because the patient usually presents with an acute and painful shoulder, inflammation is targeted before strengthening is even addressed. Nonsteroidal oral medication can help with this and should be taken for a sustained amount of time and at the correct antiinflammatory dosage, balancing the inherent risks of nonsteroidal antiinflammatory drug (NSAID) administration.[18]

Activity modification can also help decrease the pain, and once this is accomplished, a course of physical therapy focusing on range of motion exercises can be

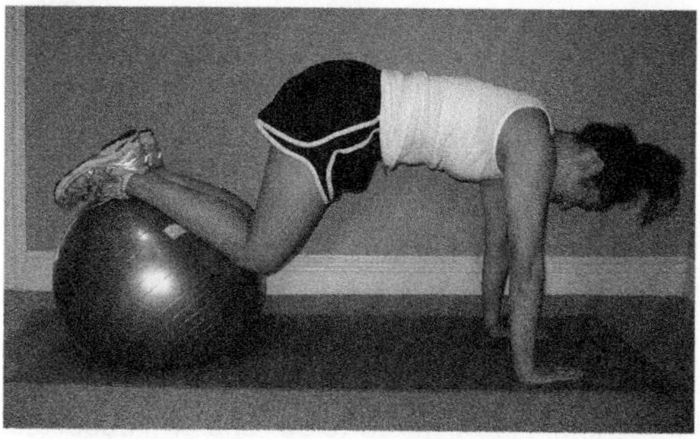

Fig. 6. Hand plank-to-tuck; knee extension and flexion on Swiss ball, strengthening core.

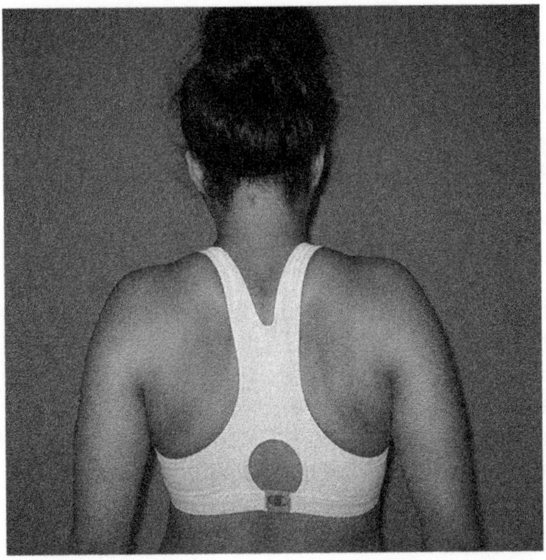

Fig. 7. Scapular set; isometric strengthening for middle/lower trapezius; scapulae retracted to midline.

started. At first, wall walking, towel-aided stretches, and use of a pulley can be integrated,[19] while avoiding abduction and overhead exercises, which exacerbate the symptoms in the early phase of rehabilitation. Once a full range of motion has been achieved, including stretching of the posterior capsule (**Fig. 10**), strength work targeting the scapular stabilizers and the rotator cuff can be incorporated (**Figs. 11** and **12**).[19] Another method of pain management used by physical therapists can be moist heat in conjunction with high-voltage electric stimulation for a period of 15 to 20 minutes per session.[20]

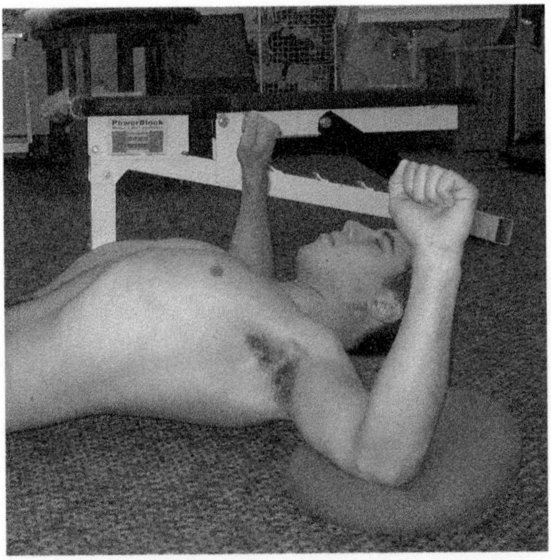

Fig. 8. Scapular strengthening; elbow flexed to 90° and arm abducted, lifting upper torso off the ground.

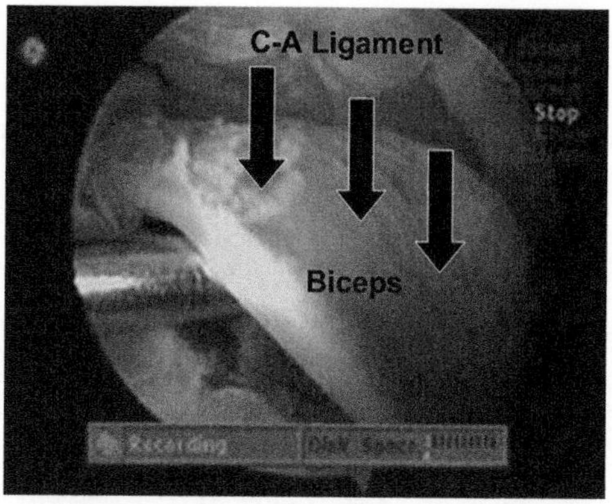

Fig. 9. Arthroscopic view of right biceps tenosynovitis (*arrows*); biceps is pulled up and out of the groove.

Subacromial injections have been used to treat primary biceps tendonitis.[21] However, there are certain guidelines to be followed when deciding to take this route. Yamaguchi and Bindra[18] administer injections only when the patient experiences continuous night pain and fails to improve during 6 weeks of treatment. These authors suggest that because biceps tendonitis may not respond to subacromial injection, better results may be achieved by direct injection into the glenohumeral joint.[18] There is also the concern for steroid-induced atrophic tendon changes; thus, peritendinous tendon sheath injection should be the objective instead of intratendinous injection.[18] To avoid injecting the tendon, Eakin and colleagues[22] recommend that the patient be placed in a sitting or supine position with 90° flexion of the elbow and the arm internally rotated 10°. The injection should be made into the area of maximum tenderness, and there should be no resistance upon injection because any needle opposition would mean intratendinous penetration. Habermeyer and Walch[23] support a single intra-articular injection of cortisone along with antiinflammatory medication during the acute phase.

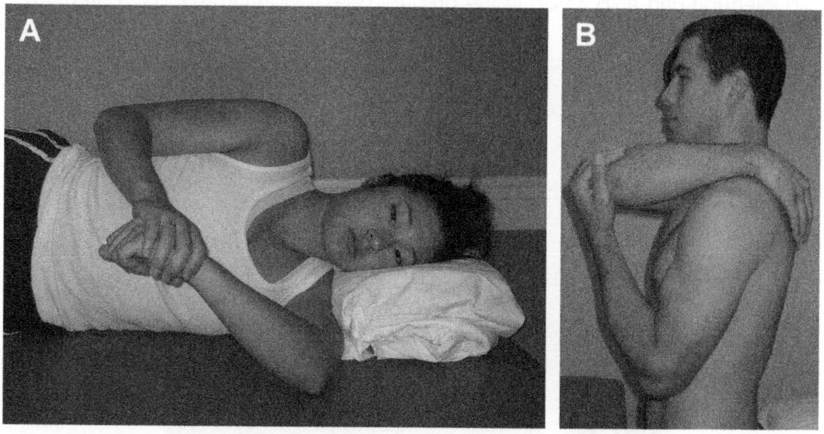

Fig. 10. (*A*) Sleeper stretch. Side lying with scapula stabilized to achieve increased internal rotation. (*B*) Horizontal adduction; cross-body adduction stretching the posterior shoulder.

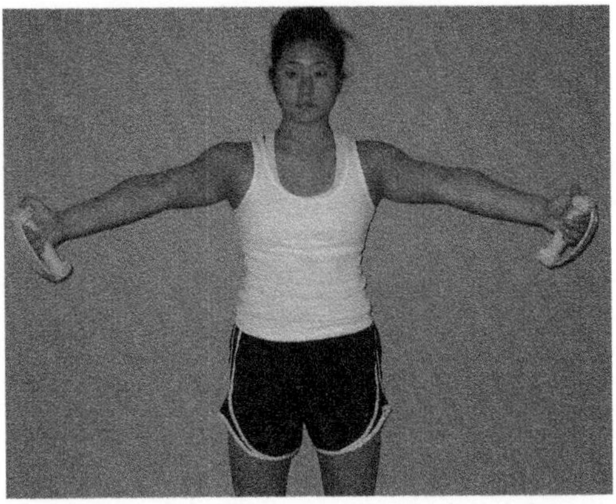

Fig. 11. Standing "scaption"; thumbs pointing up strengthens the anterosuperior rotator cuff.

As a variation of primary tendonitis, Boileau and colleagues[24] described the "hourglass" deformity of the proximal biceps tendon, which is comparable to the trigger finger phenomenon. The long head of the biceps tendon can be deformed as a result of chronic inflammatory change and may become entrapped within the joint, generating pain and locking of the shoulder with attempted elevation of the extremity. The reported cases required either a tenotomy or a tenodesis. Successful conservative management of this pathology has not been described in the literature.

Biceps Tendonitis Associated with Impingement

Secondary biceps tendonitis occurs as a result of associated shoulder pathology, such as impingement.[21] With chronic inflammation and rotator cuff fatigue, loss of humeral head containment can increase subacromial contact forces, including to the biceps. Relieving pain and restoring a balanced rotator cuff and scapula assist in maintaining a centered humeral head and a functional improvement in subacromial space clearance. The conservative treatment for secondary bicipital tendonitis is similar to that of primary tendonitis. Rest, ice, nonsteroidal medications, and physical therapy are all indicated as the first line of treatment. The judicious use of subacromial steroid injection can also assist in the primary phase of inflammation abatement.

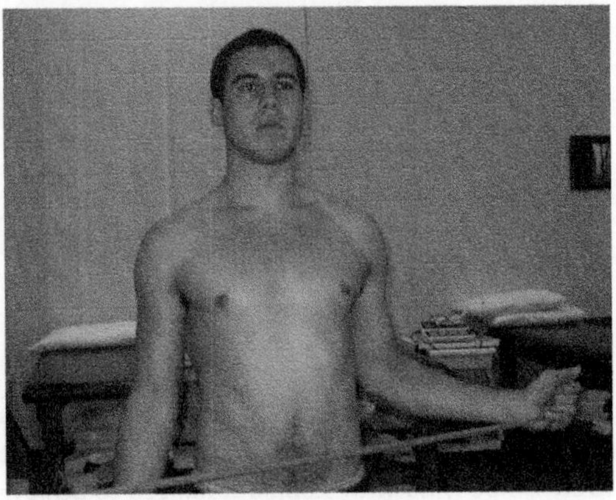

Fig. 12. Elastic band external rotation strengthening.

In a study conducted by Morrison and colleagues,[25] the physical therapy program specifically addressed the extrinsic theory (coracoacromial arch moving toward the cuff and biceps) of impingement syndrome. The rehabilitation protocol included exercises for the rotator cuff, with the arm at the side to avoid strengthening of the deltoid and to target the strength of the inferior portion of the rotator cuff. The logic behind the program being that an overstrengthened deltoid elevates the humerus, especially in the presence of a weakened cuff, thereby precipitating acromial impingement. Of the 413 patients included in the study, 67% had a satisfactory result with conservative management and 28% went on to surgery. Eighteen percent of the patients with a successful result because of conservative treatment experienced a reoccurrence of symptoms within a year.[25] However, these symptoms went away with rest or recommencement of the physical therapy protocol.[25] Senbursa and colleagues[26] found that patients treated with a joint and soft tissue mobilization regimen that included manual therapy showed more improvement than those treated with a self-guided rehabilitation program. The therapeutic exercise programs in the trial studied by Michener and colleagues[27] included stretching of the anterior and posterior shoulder girdle, muscle relaxation techniques, motor learning to normalize dysfunctional patterns of motion, and rotator cuff and scapular strengthening, all of which led to improvements in shoulder pain. Patients who underwent therapeutic exercise in combination with manual therapy techniques had the best outcome.

Though impingement is often treated conservatively, in their 2003 systematic review, Desmeules and coworkers[28] found that there was not enough evidence in the literature to support or invalidate the effectiveness of physical therapy interventions for this pathology. Treatments, such as therapeutic exercise and orthopedic manual therapy, have not been well studied, whereas more marginal therapies, such as electromagnetic field therapy and low-level laser therapy, have been.[28] Despite laser therapy not being common practice in the United States, some studies have demonstrated a short-term benefit for pain, function, and range of motion in comparison with placebo and nonsteroidals. It has been postulated that laser therapy is best used in patients who are unable to exercise.[29] With ultrasound, the limited amount of information does not support its efficacy for the treatment of subacromial impingement.[27,30]

Instability of the Biceps

Nonsurgical treatment of biceps tendon instability has not been well studied,[18] and because this instability requires a structural deficit to be corrected, nonoperative management has not been advocated.

There are several instances in which biceps instability can occur: a rotator interval deficiency, a torn or stretched medial sling (composed of the coracohumeral and superior glenohumeral ligaments) (**Figs. 13** and **14**), a subscapularis tear as well as tearing of the lateral expansion of the coracohumeral ligament and anterior edge of the supraspinatus tendon. These allow the biceps to subluxate or dislocate medially in most cases (**Fig. 15**). However, lateral subluxation can occur when the lateral expansion of the coracohumeral ligament is compromised. Suffice it to say that biceps instability, although feasible as an isolated phenomenon, is almost always associated with a rotator cuff tear.[22] The medial dislocation of the biceps, the most common instability pattern, is usually associated with a torn subscapularis tendon. Eventually, the biceps dislocates into an intra-articular position as the subscapularis retracts. In the rare case in which the biceps dislocates medially and the subscapularis is intact, the biceps can dislocate into an extra-articular position anterior to subscapularis tendon.[31]

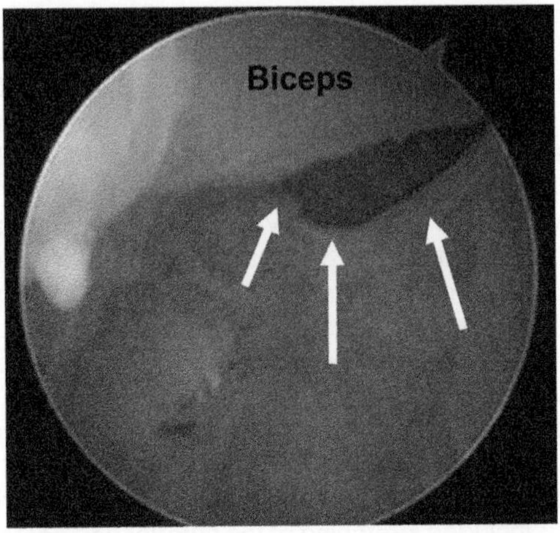

Fig. 13. Elongated (pathologic) medial sling (*arrows*) in a right shoulder.

According to some physicians, conservative treatment for biceps instability can be similar to that undertaken for biceps tendonitis, with the focus on improving rotator cuff function.[18,19] A recommendation of conservative treatment may be satisfactory in the older patient; however, there are no studies supporting this approach.

Spontaneous Rupture

Indications for the repair of biceps tendon ruptures are controversial because a nonsurgical approach can lead to very good results in the middle-aged to older patient. Spontaneous rupture is most common in this age group because they have cumulative risk and injury of the biceps tendon and rotator cuff related to overuse, attrition, and mechanical impingement.[4,32,33] Rupture frequently transpires at the proximal bicipital groove. The trauma required for rupture can often be trivial. Most of the time, chronic pain is relieved once the complete rupture has occurred as tension on the remaining fibers is released.

Although younger, more active patients may select surgical intervention,[12] studies have shown that conservative treatment of biceps rupture can lead to satisfactory function. In 1967, Carroll and Hamilton[34] studied 100 patients with a rupture of the

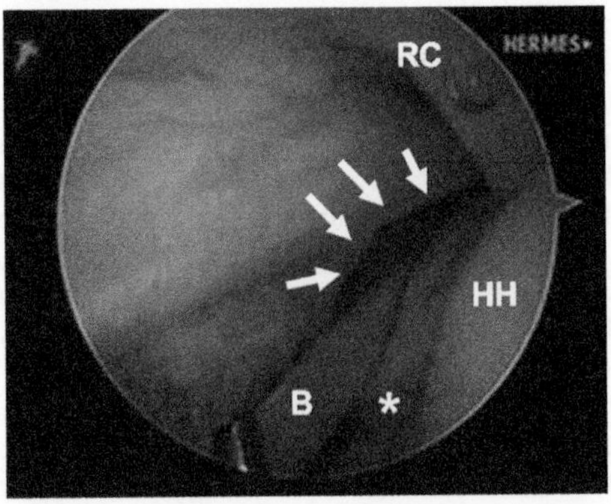

Fig. 14. Elongated medial sling (*arrows*) with biceps (B) dislocated on top of the intact subscapularis (*asterisk*) in the right shoulder. HH, humeral head; RC, rotator cuff.

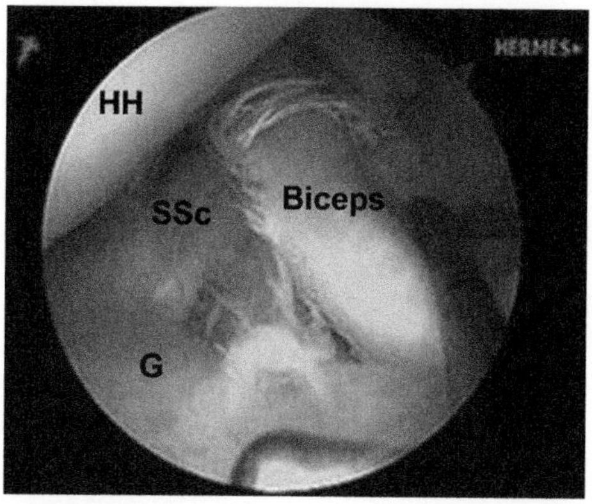

Fig. 15. Intra-articular proximal biceps dislocation in a left shoulder. HH, humeral head; G, glenoid; SSc, subscapularis.

biceps and determined that patients treated conservatively did not have any residual disability. Phillips and colleagues[35] showed that in the middle-aged or older patient, there was neither significant loss of flexion or supination abilities nor significant difference between the nonoperative group and those who underwent a tenodesis. Mariani and colleagues[36] found an 8% loss of supination in the surgical repair group and a loss of 21% forearm supination strength in patients who did not undergo surgery. There was no significant difference between the elbow flexion strength of the 2 groups. Furthermore, those treated nonoperatively returned to work sooner.

However, Meyer[37] demonstrated that if the long head of the biceps tendon was left unrepaired, there was a 21% loss of supination ability and an 8% to 20% loss of elbow flexion strength in comparison with those people who opted to have surgical treatment. Thus, if supination, such as using a screwdriver, is important in a patient's line of work, surgery could be indicated regardless of age. A conservative approach is appropriate if the patient is not extremely active, does not mind some loss of arm strength, and has a potential for a cosmetic deformity. Thus, conservative treatment of the biceps rupture in the elderly population is advocated by many physicians, and few patients in this age bracket have significant problems related to the biceps rupture itself.[4] The strength deficit that may result from a biceps tendon rupture can be compensated for, and the loss of muscle strength after rupture has been postulated to be less than 20%.[38] Sometimes in the case of an elderly patient, the diseased biceps tendon is flatter and broader (**Fig. 16**), requiring a greater force to pull it through the bicipital groove,[39] thereby creating its own durable fixation strength or autotenodesis.

The 2 most common complaints with conservative management of proximal biceps tendon rupture are upper arm deformity and cramping with strenuous activities (**Fig. 17**). Aside from the cosmetic issue, the cramping usually subsides with time, although some may complain of intermittent episodes on a long-term basis associated with vigorous repetitive elbow flexion. Activity modification rather than physical therapy is the most effective management for this symptom.

POSTOPERATIVE REHABILITATION

Surgical Treatment

Surgery for proximal biceps disease is predicated on causation. Although surgical management of biceps tendon pathology is not always the definitive solution, arthroscopic rather than open treatment of these lesions is becoming the preferred method.

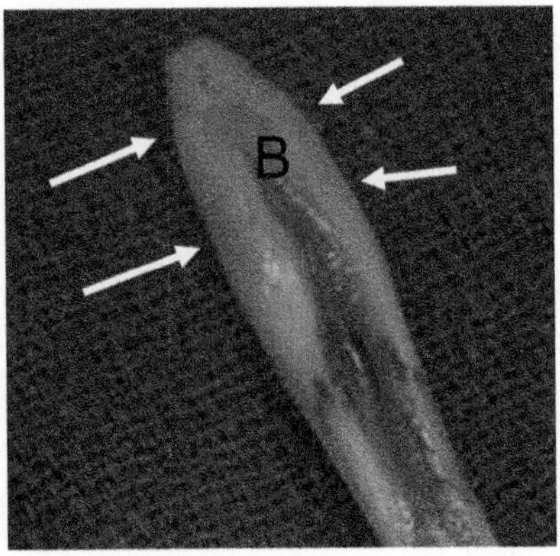

Fig. 16. Chronically thickened (*arrows*) and inflamed proximal biceps (B) tendon.

Surgery is usually indicated in those patients with symptomatic biceps instability, with or without concomitant rotator cuff disease. In patients with primary or secondary biceps tendonitis resistant to conservative measures, arthroscopic intervention in the form of a tenodesis or tenotomy may be indicated.[40]

Tenotomy

Biceps tenotomy has been advocated for patients with biceps tendonitis alone or in conjunction with a rotator cuff tear.[41] The advantages of a tenotomy are (1) technical simplicity, (2) shorter and less complex rehabilitation time, and (3) accelerated return to daily activities. However, tenotomies are associated with "Popeye" deformity, which may be cosmetically unappealing and can be associated with muscle weakness and cramping with vigorous activities.[42] Tenotomy has been recommended for older, less active individuals,[40] and has been associated with a high satisfaction rate with regard to pain relief.

Tenodesis

Although a more complex surgical intervention than tenotomy, treatment by tenodesis (open or arthroscopic) maintains the length-tension relationship[39] and minimizes the

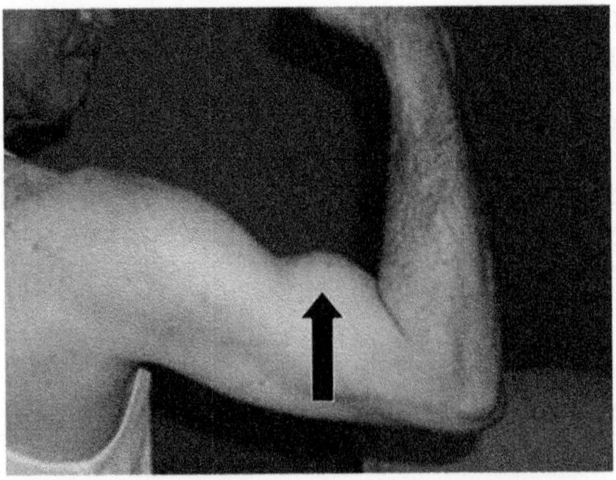

Fig. 17. Popeye deformity (*arrow*). Lateral view of exaggerated distal biceps after spontaneous rupture and distal retraction.

loss of flexion and supination ability while lessening the risk of postoperative cramping and Popeye deformity.[40] The indications for biceps tenodesis are (1) significant tearing of the biceps tendon; (2) medial subluxation, with or without a torn subscapularis tendon[43]; and (3) symptomatic SLAP lesions in the older population or in conjunction with a rotator cuff repair.

Although there are advantages and disadvantages for both procedures, a significant difference in outcome has not been detected.[44] Failure rates for tenodesis range from 5%[45] to 48%[46] and for tenotomy, from 13%[41] to 35%.[47]

Biomechanics and Rehabilitation After Tenotomy

Postoperative rehabilitation after simple tenotomy can be more aggressive because minimal protection is needed for the healing tissue.[48] The greatest risk to this approach is the development of the Popeye deformity. The phenomenon has been reported in 62% to 70% of patients after tenotomy.[49] After this procedure, patients potentially have an unrestricted range of motion, and their return to activities is limited only by their symptoms[12] because there is no need for postoperative immobilization.[40]

Knowing the strength of tendon scarring after tenotomy can help predict the possibility of a distal deformity. In a biomechanical study comparing pullout-strength values after a release of the biceps, Bradbury and colleagues[42] found the mean force required to pull the tendon through the bicipital groove to be 25 N (5.62 lb) if the biceps was released without a portion of the superior labrum and 73.2 N (16.45 lb) if it was released with a portion of the superior labrum equal to twice the width of the biceps tendon and half the height of the superior labrum. The rationale behind this difference was presumed wedging of the proximal biceps stump into the opening of the bicipital groove. In a study conducted by Wolf and colleagues,[50] the mean load to failure after tenotomy was 110.7 N (24.88 lb). Wolf and colleagues[50] theorized that with an ultimate load to failure of 110 N, minimal resistance (approximately 5 lb) held in the hand would lead to distal migration of the tendon and cosmetic deformity.

Even though the patients are allowed to return to their activities quickly after tenotomy, there is still a concern about tendon migration due to stress on the biceps tendon. Post-tenotomy patients should not lift heavy objects or do weight training right after surgery because of the possibility of distal migration and a less pleasing esthetic result. If the objectives are wedging and tissue healing within the groove, it probably makes sense to delay extremely vigorous activity for a few months after tenotomy (although there is no compelling evidence in this regard).

Biomechanics After Tenodesis

A more sophisticated program than rehabilitation after tenotomy is required after tenodesis. Wolf and colleagues[50] determined that the mean load to failure after tenodesis was 310.8 N in contrast to the 110 N after tenotomy. They concluded that gentle early postoperative range of motion was safe without risk of distal tendon migration. Mazzocca and colleagues[51] investigated 4 different fixation techniques, including subpectoral bone tunnel (SBT), arthroscopic interference screw (AIS), subpectoral interference screw (SIS), and arthroscopic suture anchor (SA) technique to compare the strength of each construct (axial load to failure) and to determine whether the construct could withstand an accelerated rehabilitation protocol (cyclic displacement). In regard to cyclic displacement, there was no significant difference between the AIS, SIS, and SA techniques; however, the SBT demonstrated less favorable results. All 4 techniques had favorable load to failure characteristics: SIS (252 N), SBT (242 N), AIS (237 N), and SA (164 N).[51] Golish and coworkers[52] found that an interference screw construct (169.9 N) had a higher ultimate load to failure than suture anchor fixation (68.5 N) when used for tenodesis in a subpectoral location.

In another study, Ozalay and colleagues[53] showed in a sheep model that interference screw fixation (243 N) was superior to bone tunnel fixation (229 N), suture anchor fixation (129 N), and the keyhole technique (101 N). Although their results did not fully corroborate the findings of Mazzocca, in both studies interference screw fixation of the biceps tendon was the superior construct. Ozalay and colleagues concluded that the satisfactory pullout strength of the interference screw technique permits an accelerated rehabilitation program in which minimal immobilization was required and early range of motion could be initiated. It is noteworthy that although Ozalay and colleagues found keyhole tenodesis to be the weakest fixation, the study by Jayamoorthy and colleagues[32] found keyhole tenodesis (303 N) to be stronger than interference screw (234 N) and metallic screw (210 N) techniques. They argued that keyhole tenodesis should also be considered by surgeons because of its strong fixation strength. The differences between the studies may be reflected in bone quality, origin of the specimen, and permutations in the loading protocol.

Based on the biomechanical studies that evaluate pullout strength after tenodesis, patients may be treated in a simple sling for comfort for a few weeks while avoiding vigorous flexion and supination to prevent compromising the repair.[12]

Tendon Healing

The rate at which the biceps tendon heals after tenodesis determines the timeline of postoperative rehabilitation. Healing may take up to 12 weeks and is therefore the key factor to be considered in an accelerated rehab program. To achieve secure tendon-to-bone healing, Rodeo and colleagues[54] determined in the canine model that tendon-to-bone healing required approximately 12 weeks. Although biceps tenodesis was not studied specifically, one can extrapolate that a soft tissue–bone tenodesis should be protected for up to 12 weeks. Rodeo and colleagues[54] also noted that the greatest gains in strength of the repair occurred during the first 4 weeks. Clearly, if tendon fixation is stressed prematurely, the repair may fail. Some rehabilitation programs initiate resistive exercises at approximately 6 weeks postoperatively.[12,18] This seems to contradict the healing process that Rodeo and colleagues discussed, and in patients for whom the return to sport or activity is absolutely imperative without risk of failure, mandating a few more weeks for healing time may be ideal.

The exact sequence and quantification of tendon-to-bone healing for the long head of the biceps in the initial 3 months after repair are currently unknown. Gerber and colleagues[55] ascertained in the sheep model that the load to failure of an infraspinatus tendon was 30% of that of a normal tendon at 6 weeks, 52% at 3 months, and 81% at 6 months. The slow rate of tendon healing can potentially be explained by the decrease of blood flow as the tendon enters the bicipital groove and the resultant low oxygen tension, which is 7.5 times lower than that recorded in skeletal muscle.

Forces generated during rehabilitation should not exceed the pullout strength. It requires approximately 112 N to maintain the weight of the forearm at 90° while holding a 2.2-lb object.[56] It has been estimated that the force on the biceps tendon is 75 N while supporting the weight of the forearm against gravity and up to 300 N with a 4.5-lb object held in the hand.[32]

Rehabilitation Exercises

At this point, there is no preferred rehabilitation program after tenodesis and tenotomy based on evidence-based medicine. One can guide the protocol only based on a solid understanding of the basic science of tissue healing. The rehabilitation programs currently recommended are designed for postoperative rotator cuff tears and are inclusive of the biceps. Yamaguchi and Bindra[18] follow rotator cuff guidelines for their patients with tenodesis. They restrict resisted flexion and supination for 6 weeks, moving from early passive range of motion immediately after surgery and progressing to active assisted and then active. Burkhead and colleagues[4] immobilize the arm for 3 weeks postoperatively. The patient starts with gentle passive pendulum exercises on the first postoperative day and passive flexion on the second. At 1 month, a pulley is used for active elbow flexion, whereas strengthening of the rotator cuff, deltoid, and biceps begins at 2 months with more vigorous activity allowed at 3 months.

SUMMARY

The function of the biceps continues to be an enigma. Although proximal biceps injuries remain uncommon in young people, tearing or instability can occur and are more frequent in the older population. Specific testing during physical examination correlated with diagnostic imaging usually helps to pinpoint the diagnosis. Conservative management of biceps pathology is typically the first line of treatment, including measures such as rest, activity modification, ice, NSAIDs, physical therapy, and potentially steroid injection. Failed improvement in the pain level may be an indication for surgical intervention. Often, diagnostic arthroscopy becomes the best method for determining and treating the pathology. Tenotomy and tenodesis are the most common surgical procedures for remedying proximal biceps dysfunction. Post-tenotomy or post-tenodesis rehabilitation protocols are different because of distinct differences in tendon biomechanics. The physician must also be aware of the physiology of postsurgical repair and advocate appropriate rehabilitation activities that correlate with the timeline of secure tissue healing.

REFERENCES

1. Vangsness CT Jr, Jorgenson SS, Watson T, et al. The origin of the long head of the biceps from the scapula and glenoid labrum. An anatomical study of 100 shoulders. J Bone Joint Surg Br 1994;76:951–4.
2. Alpantaki K, McLaughlin D, Karagogoes D, et al. Sympathetic and sensory neural elements in the tendon of the long head of the biceps. J Bone Joint Surg Am 2005;87:1580–3.
3. Habermeyer P, Magosch P, Pritsch M, et al. Anterosuperior impingement of the shoulder as a result of pulley impingement of the shoulder as a result of pulley lesions: a prospective arthroscopic study. J Shoulder Elbow Surg 2004;13:5–12.
4. Burkhead WZ, Arcand MA, Zeman C, et al. The biceps tendon. In: Rockwood CA, Matsen FA, Wirth MA, et al, editors. The shoulder, vol. 2. 3rd edition. Philadelphia: WB Saunders; 2004. p. 1059–115.
5. Barber FA, Field LD, Ryu RKN. Biceps tendon and superior labrum injuries: decision-making. J Bone Joint Surg Am 2007;89:1844–55.
6. Altchek D, Wolf B. Disorders of the biceps tendon. In: Krishnan S, Hawkins R, Warren R, editors. The shoulder and the overhead athlete. Philadelphia: Lippincott Williams & Wilkins; 2004. p. 196–208.
7. Sethi N, Wright R, Yamaguchi K. Disorders of the long head of the biceps tendon. J Shoulder Elbow Surg 1999;8(6):644–54.
8. Rodosky MW, Harder CD, Fu F. The role of the long head of the biceps muscle and superior glenoid labrum in anterior stability of the shoulder. Am J Sports Med 1994;22(1):121–30.

9. Krupp RJ, Kevern MA, Gaines MD, et al. Long head of the biceps tendon pain: differential diagnosis and treatment. J Orthop Sports Phys Ther 2009;39(2): 55–68.
10. Krishnan SG, Hawkins RJ, Bokor D. Clinical evaluation of shoulder problems. In: Rockwood CA, Matsen FA, Wirth MA, et al, editors. The shoulder. 3rd edition. Philadelphia: WB Saunders; 2004.
11. Yergason RM. Supination sign. J Bone Joint Surg 1931;131:60.
12. Hsu SH, Miller SL, Curtis AS. Long head of biceps tendon pathology: management alternatives. Clin Sports Med 2008;27(4):747–62.
13. Green S, Buchbinder R, Hetrick S. Physiotherapy interventions for shoulder pain. Cochrane Database Syst Rev 2003;(2):CD004258.
14. DePalma AF. The painful shoulder. Postgrad Med 1957;21:368–76.
15. Favorito PJ, Harding WG 3rd, Heidt RS Jr. Complete arthroscopic examination of the long head of the biceps tendon. Arthroscopy 2001;17(4):430–2.
16. Ruotolo C, Nottage WM, Flatow EL, et al. Controversial topics in shoulder arthroscopy. Arthroscopy 2002;18(2):65–75.
17. Post D, Benca P. Primary tendonitis of the long head of the biceps. Clin Orthop Relat Res 1989;246:117–25.
18. Yamaguchi K, Bindra R. Disorders of the biceps tendon. In: Iannotti JP, Williams GR, editors. Disorders of the shoulder: diagnosis and management. Philadelphia: Lippincott Williams & Wilkins; 1999. p. 159–89.
19. Paynter KS. Disorders of the long head of the biceps tendon. Phys Med Rehabil Clin N Am 2004;15(2):511–28.
20. Ellenbecker TS, Derscheid GL. Rehabilitation of overuse injuries of the shoulder. Clin Sports Med 1989;8(3):583–603.
21. Nevaiser RJ. Lesions of the biceps and tendinitis of the shoulder. Orthop Clin North Am 1980;11:343–8.
22. Eakin CL, Faber KL, Hawkins RJ. Biceps tendon disorders in athletes. J Am Acad Orthop Surg 1999;7(5):300–10.
23. Habermeyer P, Walch G. The biceps tendon and rotator cuff disease. In: Burkhead WZ, editor. Rotator cuff disorders. Media (PA): Lippincott Williams & Wilkins; 1996. p. 142.
24. Boileau P, Ahrens PM, Hatzidakis AM. Entrapment of the long head of the biceps tendon: the hourglass biceps—a cause of pain and locking of the shoulder. J Shoulder Elbow Surg 2004;13(3):249–57.
25. Morrison DS, Frogameni AD, Woodworth P. Non-operative treatment of subacromial impingement syndrome. J Bone Joint Surg Am 1997;79:732–7.
26. Senbursa G, Baltaci G, Atay A. Comparison of conservative treatment with or without manual physical therapy for patients with shoulder impingement syndrome: a prospective, randomized clinical trial. Knee Surg Sports Traumatol Arthrosc 2007;15(7):915–21.
27. Michener LA, Walsworth MK, Burnet EN. Effectiveness of rehabilitation for patients with subacromial impingement syndrome: a systematic review. J Hand Ther 2004;17(2):152–64.
28. Desmeules F, Cote CH, Fremont P. Therapeutic exercise and orthopedic manual therapy for impingement syndrome: a systematic review. Clin J Sport Med 2003; 13:176–82.
29. England S, Farrell AJ, Coppock JS, et al. Low power laser therapy of shoulder tendonitis. Scand J Rheumatol 1989;18:427–31.
30. Sauers EL. Effectiveness of rehabilitation for patients with subacromial impingement syndrome. J Athl Train 2005;40(3):221–3.

31. Tonino PM, Gerber C, Itoi E, et al. Complex shoulder disorders: evaluation and treatment. J Am Acad Orthop Surg 2009;17(3):125–36.
32. Jayamoorthy T, Field JR, Costi JJ, et al. Biceps tenodesis: a biomechanical study of fixation methods. J Shoulder Elbow Surg 2004;13(2):160–4.
33. Neer CS 2nd. Anterior acromioplasty for the chronic impingement syndrome in the shoulder: a preliminary report. J Bone Joint Surg Am 1972;54(1):41–50.
34. Carroll RE, Hamilton LR. Rupture of the biceps brachii—a conservative method of treatment. J Bone Joint Surg Am 1967;49:1016.
35. Phillips BB, Canale ST, Sisk TD, et al. Ruptures of the proximal biceps tendon in middle-aged patients. Orthop Rev 1993;22(3):349–53.
36. Mariani EM, Cofield RM, Askew LJ, et al. Rupture of the tendon of the long head of the biceps brachii: surgical versus nonsurgical treatment. Clin Orthop Relat Res 1986;228:233–9.
37. Meyer AW. Unrecognized occupational destruction of the tendon of the long head of the biceps brachii. Arch Surg 1921;2:130–44.
38. Sturzenegger M, Beguin D, Grunig B, et al. Muscular strength after rupture of the long head of the biceps. Arch Orthop Trauma Surg 1986;105:18–23.
39. Ahmad CS, DiSipio C, Lester J. Factors affecting dropped biceps deformity after tenotomy of the long head of the biceps tendon. Arthroscopy 2007;23(5):537–41.
40. Friedman DJ, Dunn JC, Higgins LD. Proximal biceps tendon: injuries and management. Sports Med Arthrosc 2008;16(3):162–9.
41. Gill TJ, McIrvin E, Mair SD, et al. Results of biceps tenotomy for treatment of pathology of the long head of the biceps brachii. J Shoulder Elbow Surg 2001; 10(3):247–9.
42. Bradbury T, Dunn WR, Kuhn JE. Preventing the popeye deformity after release of the long head of the biceps tendon: an alternative technique and biomechanical evaluation. Arthroscopy 2008;24(10):1099–102.
43. Richards DP, Burkhart SS, Lo IK. Subscapularis tears: arthroscopic repair techniques. Orthop Clin North Am 2003;34(4):485–98.
44. Frost A, Zafar MS, Maffulli N. Tenotomy versus tenodesis in the management of pathology lesions of the tendon of the long head of the biceps brachii. Am J Sports Med 2009;37(4):828–33.
45. Boileau P, Krishnan SG, Coste JS, et al. Arthroscopic biceps tenodesis: a new technique using bioabsorbable interference screw fixation. Arthroscopy 2002; 18(9):1002–12.
46. Becker DA, Cofield RH. Tenodesis of the long head of the biceps brachii for chronic bicipital tendonitis. Long-term results. J Bone Joint Surg Am 1989;71: 376–81.
47. Kelly AM, Drakos MC, Fealy S. Arthroscopic release of the long head of the biceps tendon: functional outcome and clinical results. Am J Sports Med 2005; 33(2):208–13.
48. Ahrens PM, Boileau P. The long head of the biceps and associated tendinopathy. J Bone Joint Surg Br 2007;89(8):1001–9.
49. Boileau P, Baque F, Valerior L, et al. Isolated arthroscopic bíceps tenotomy or tenodesis improves symptoms in patients with massive irreparable rotator cuff tears. J Bone Joint Surg Am 2007;89(4):747–57.
50. Wolf RS, Zheng N, Weichel D. Long head biceps tenotomy versus tenodesis: a cadaveric analysis. Arthroscopy 2005;21(2):182–5.
51. Mazzocca AD, Bicos J, Santangelo S, et al. The biomechanical evaluation of four fixation techniques for proximal biceps tenodesis. Arthroscopy 2005;21(11): 1296–306.

52. Golish SR, Caldwell PE, Miller MD, et al. Interference screw versus suture anchor fixation for subpectoral tenodesis of the proximal biceps tendon: a cadaveric study. Arthroscopy 2008;24(10):1103–8.
53. Ozalay M, Akpinar S, Karaeminogullari O, et al. Mechanical strength of four different biceps tenodesis techniques. Arthroscopy 2005;21(8):992–8.
54. Rodeo SA, Arnoczky SP, Torzilli PA, et al. Tendon-healing in a bone tunnel. A biomechanical and histological study in the dog. J Bone Joint Surg Am 1993;75:1795–803.
55. Gerber C, Schneeberger AG, Perren SM. Experimental rotator cuff repair. A preliminary study. J Bone Joint Surg Am 1999;81(9):1281–90.
56. Verma NN. Long head biceps tendon: indications and techniques for surgical management. In: online course syllabus and presentation materials for San Diego Shoulder Institute Annual Meeting: shoulder arthroscopy, arthroplasty, fractures, June 2009. Available at: http://www.shoulder.com/.

Rehabilitation After Arthroscopic Decompression for Femoroacetabular Impingement

Keelan R. Enseki, MS, PT, ATC, OCS, SCS, CSCS[a,b,c],
RobRoy Martin, PhD, PT, CSCS[a,d], Bryan T. Kelly, MD[e,*]

KEYWORDS

- Hip • Acetabular labrum
- Femoral acetabular impingement • Rehabilitation

Diagnostic and surgical advancements have greatly expanded the treatment options available to individuals with pathologic conditions of the hip joint. Recently, increased attention has been devoted to treating the condition of femoroacetabular impingement (FAI). FAI has been suggested as playing a role in the development of acetabular labral tears and chondral lesions, which may potentially progress to more advanced degenerative changes of the hip joint.[1–9] Arthroscopic decompression has become a feasible treatment option for individuals diagnosed with FAI. The femoral or acetabular components of FAI may be addressed through this application. To optimize treatment outcomes, postoperative rehabilitation must evolve in parallel to current surgical advancements.

Postoperative rehabilitation protocols for various arthroscopic procedures of the hip joint have been described in the literature.[10,11] The majority of these protocols have focused heavily on procedures involving débridement or repair of the acetabular labrum. Additional considerations are often suggested for cases that involve additional procedures, including capsular modification (plication or capsulorrhaphy), tendon release (iliopsoas or iliotibial band), microfracture procedures and other cartilage preservation procedures, and decompression for FAI (femoral or acetabular components).

[a] Centers for Rehab Services, Center for Sports Medicine, University of Pittsburgh, Pittsburgh, PA, USA
[b] Department of Physical Therapy, University of Pittsburgh, Pittsburgh, PA, USA
[c] Department of Sports Medicine and Nutrition, University of Pittsburgh, Pittsburgh, PA, USA
[d] Department of Physical Therapy, Duquesne University, Pittsburgh, PA, USA
[e] Hospital for Special Surgery, 535 East 70th Street, New York, NY 10021, USA
* Corresponding author.
E-mail address: kellyb@hss.edu (B.T. Kelly).

Clin Sports Med 29 (2010) 247–255
doi:10.1016/j.csm.2009.12.007 **sportsmed.theclinics.com**
0278-5919/10/$ – see front matter

Traditional postoperative protocols for hip surgery procedures (primarily arthroplasty procedures) are not entirely applicable to individuals undergoing arthroscopic decompression procedures to address FAI. These protocols do not suffice for several reasons. The arthroscopic approach does not involve dislocation of the hip joint that is used in the majority of open procedures. Therefore, traditional range-of-motion (ROM) precautions to avoid postoperative dislocation are not necessary. Additionally, the characteristics of population likely to undergo arthroscopic decompression vary from those likely to receive arthroplasty procedures. Individuals undergoing arthroscopy to address FAI are likely to originate from a more physically active population. Secondary to these reasons, the postoperative rehabilitation approach described more closely resembles a modified postoperative arthroscopic labral débridement protocol as opposed to a modified hip arthroplasty rehabilitation protocol.

Rehabilitation for individuals undergoing arthroscopic decompression to address FAI should be based on the known healing properties of osseous tissues and any other tissues affected by the surgical procedure. The most critical concern is preservation of the blood supply to the neck and head of the femur. Fracture of the femoral neck and avascular necrosis of the femoral head are concerns secondary to the transient bony compromise created through surgical decompresion. The latter likely necessitates patients undergoing a joint arthroplasty procedure. In addition to concerns for weight bearing, considerations regarding early ROM restrictions are necessary. This ROM restriction is not to avoid dislocation as with hip replacement, rather, to avoid progression of inflammation from the decompressed femoral head-neck and or acetabular rim being squeezed together. Therefore, excessive hip flexion, abduction, and internal rotation are typically limited early in the rehabilitation process.

IMMEDIATE POSTOPERATIVE REHABILITATION

The goals of rehabilitation immediately after surgery are the same as the majority of other orthopedic procedures. Measures should be taken to control pain and postoperative inflammation and to provide an optimal healing environment for the joint. Nonsteroidal anti-inflammatory drugs (NSAIDs) may be prescribed at the surgeon's discretion. Ice or compression should also be used at regular intervals. Various commercial pressurized ice compression systems are commercially available and may be beneficial for patients undergoing arthroscopic surgery of the hip joint. ROM can be initially limited through the use of a postoperative brace (Bledsoe Philippon Post-Arthroscopy Hip Brace, Bledsoe Brace Systems, Grand Prairie, TX, USA) at the discretion of the surgeon. This brace limits abduction and is most often set to limit motion in the sagittal plane from neutral to approximately 80° of flexion. Patients typically use this brace during waking hours for 1 to 2 weeks. Patients may also be required to apply an immobilizer system (Bledsoe Philippon Post-Arthroscopy Hip Brace, Bledsoe Brace Systems) while sleeping. This system consists of a dense foam centerpiece with straps to immobilize the hips and not allow movement toward external rotation while patients are sleeping. Limiting external rotation limits the amount of tension placed on the anterior capsular structures. This is particularly relevant for those individuals undergoing associated capsular modification procedures. Use of the immobilizer system for patients undergoing decompression surgery for FAI has been dictated by surgeon discretion.

Patient education is a critical part of the early rehabilitation process. Optimally, patients should be aware of the time commitment and demands of rehabilitation before undergoing arthroscopy. If not addressed preoperatively, patients should be educated to ambulate correctly with crutches according to the assigned weight-bearing status. Many patients have the expectation of returning to a relatively high level of activity after surgery. For this reason, the rehabilitation process may be involved. The total time from surgery to address FAI to return to high-level activity is rarely less than 12 weeks. There may be rare exceptions to this estimate of time. Time frame for return to physically demanding activity should not be shorter than the required time for tissue healing, however. Failure to adhere to this principle may result in postoperative complications.

Immediate postoperative therapeutic activities are relatively gentle with the goal of maintaining joint ROM, circulation, and muscle integrity without prolonging the inflammatory process. Gentle passive ROM, ankle and knee muscle contraction exercises, and isometric hip muscle contraction activities are used. The stationary bike is used as soon as tolerated by the patient. Initially, the resistance should be minimal and the seat kept at a relatively high setting to avoid excessive flexion. Initial exercises may include: active ankle plantarflexion, isometric quadriceps setting, isometric gluteal setting, and posterior pelvic tilt exercises.

WEIGHT-BEARING PROGRESSION

The primary goals of limiting the weight-bearing status of patient status post arthroscopic decompression to address FAI are to protect the vulnerable osseous tissue and provide optimal joint loading to encourage a proper healing environment. A partial weight-bearing status of approximately 20 pounds, or foot-flat, is typically assigned. Crutches are used to maintain this status. This limited weight-bearing status is typically assigned for 2 to 6 weeks depending on a variety of patient factors and surgical specifics. These factors include the amount of bone débrided, treatment of the labrum (repair vs débridement), patient body mass, and individual surgeon preference. Gradual weaning off crutches over a 1- to 2-week period is generally recommended. Individual differences in tolerance to increased weight bearing are often noted. Although general guidelines are provided, patient presentation and clinical judgment should be the principal factor in determining the rate of progression for increasing weight-bearing status.

Aquatic therapy is often useful in progressing patients' weight-bearing and ambulatory activities. The buoyant environment allows a controlled approach to gait training and safe initiation of closed chain activities. Typically, these activities are initiated in chest high water. The level of water is gradually decreased as tolerated. The aquatic environment is particularly beneficial in progression of the active/athletic population. Deweighted jogging or treading may be initiated to provide safe aerobic training well before patients are able to initiate such activities on dry land.

RANGE OF MOTION

ROM progression follows relatively basic guidelines. The first 2 weeks are considered a protective stage. ROM is initiated as tolerated with caution exerted to avoid excessive hip flexion, internal rotation, and abduction. Early excessive motion in these directions may cause inflammation of tissue in the vicinity of the joint. The amount of motion is typically guided by patients' report of discomfort. Excessive force to the femoral neck region should be avoided early in the rehabilitation process. The motion of internal rotation with the hip in a flexed position should be approached with caution. Overpressure in this position may directly engage the area of the femoral head-neck junction with the acetabulum. This can cause irritation of the healing osseous tissue and excessive torsion of the femoral neck.Once the inflammation decreases, however, full passive ROM should be encouraged. This usually occurs between 2 to 4 weeks after surgery. The recommendation of restricted motion for 2 to 4 weeks followed by progression to full flexion, internal rotation, and abduction ROM should be communicated to therapists to avoid early propagation of the inflammation and later stiffness. Stretching of the hamstrings may be initiated 2 to 3 weeks after surgery. By 4 weeks post surgery, gentle stretching of all musculature in the hip joint region should be initiated and progressed as tolerated. Patients who continue to have a pinching sensation with hip flexion may do better with weight-bearing flexion from the quadruped position (**Fig. 1**). The pinching sensation can also be decreased with the use of gentle manual caudal joint distraction during flexion (**Fig. 2**).

STRENGTH

Gentle strength activities are initiated the day after surgery. These previously mentioned activities are primarily submaximal lower extremity isometrics and gentle AROM. Progression of strength activities usually begins 2 weeks after surgery. The gluteus medius muscle is of particular interest. Non–weight-bearing activities are initially used and exclusively continued until patients' weight-bearing status permits weight-bearing activities. Individuals undergoing concomitant procedures to release the iliotibial band or iliposoas tendon should delay the initiation of specific straight leg raise activities to avoid irritation of healing tissue. For those patients having the iliotibial band released, side-lying abduction should be deferred for approximately 4 weeks. Patients having the iliopsoas tendon released should avoid initiation of straight leg raises in supine. Initiation of these activities too early in the rehabilitation process may result in postoperative tendonitis. In a side-lying clamshell (patient lies on nonsurgical side and lifts knee without raising foot) or sitting position, short lever hip flexion may be used before transitioning to traditional straight leg raise exercises.

Weight-bearing strengthening activities are typically initiated 4 to 6 weeks after surgery. General strength activities should focus on the quadriceps, hamstrings, and gluteal muscle groups. Strengthening activities that involve movement in the transverse plain should not be neglected. Clinicians should monitor patients closely for signs of increased irritation. As patients progress, an emphasis should be placed on functional activities. The authors find regaining gluteus medius strength is critical

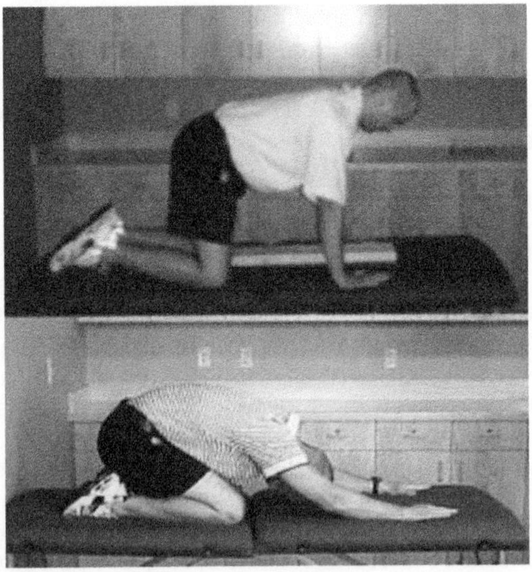

Fig. 1. Flexion performed from the quadruped position.

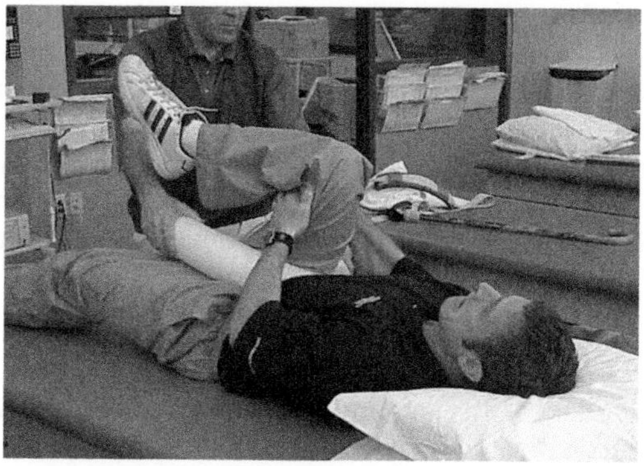

Fig. 2. The therapist produces a caudal glide of the femur while the subject uses their upper extremities to pull the hip into a flexed position.

to allowing patients to progress with single-limb support exercises. Therapists need to emphasize gluteus medius exercises early to facilitate frontal plane pelvic stability necessary for single-limb support activities.

It is common for patients with hip pathologic conditions of the hip joint to report a history of lumbopelvic complex dysfunction. Common issues include lumbopelvic instability and sacroiliac joint dysfunction. Lumbopelvic stabilization exercises are an integral part of the postoperative rehabilitation protocol. Potential exercises include pelvic tilts, bridging, extremity extension with pelvic stabilization, and abdominal isometrics. Much as scapulothoracic stabilization is needed for proper upper extremity function, lumbopelvic stabilization is required for proper lower extremity function.

FUNCTIONAL PROGRESSION

The majority of individuals undergoing arthroscopic decompression for FAI are active people. Postoperative rehabilitation programs must include the appropriate progression of functional activities to be comprehensive. Balance activities should be initiated as tolerated once tolerance to bearing full weight is established. Specific functional exercises should be dictated by the patient's goals and the specific demands of their normal activities.

Initiation of endurance activities is guided by the amount of impact and other physical demands involved. Weight-bearing endurance activities (elliptical or stepper machines) are often initiated at approximately 6 to 8 weeks after surgery. A gradual jogging progression is typically allowed approximately 12 weeks after surgery. A subpopulation of individuals may have known cartilage issues or focal areas of degeneration. A cross-training approach, using a combination of aerobic exercise activities, may prove beneficial for these patients. This approach may reduce the rate of additional cartilage degeneration. Patient education in joint protection strategies is an important component in providing complete care for this group of individuals. The authors find restoring gluteus medius and lumbopelvic stabilization critical to the success of the functional activity progression.

RETURN TO ACTIVITY

Many factors play a role in determining the return to specific activities. The demands of an individual's specific activities, physical characteristics, tissues affected by surgery, and performance in previous stages of rehabilitation all moderate the time before being allowed to return to previous activities. Manual laborers may be allowed to return to work in 12 to 24 weeks. Athletes may return to the competitive environment in 12 to 32 weeks. In rare cases, earlier return is possible. The time of return should not be sooner than the time frame of healing for the tissues affected by surgery, however. Before being allowed to resume strenuous physical activity, patients should achieve appropriate ROM, flexibility, strength, and endurance. In addition, patients should demonstrate satisfactory performance on functional testing of ability to withstand the rigors of specific occupational or athletic demands.

POSTOPERATIVE REHABILITATION COMPLICATIONS

Through clinical experience, the authors have noted several recurrent issues that occur during the rehabilitation process in the population of patients undergoing arthroscopic decompression to address FAI. The majority of these occurrences can be avoided with careful monitoring of patients' symptom presentation and adherence to the basic principles of postoperative rehabilitation protocols. Once present, these complications may be difficult to address. Often, a significant decrease of activities required to return patients' symptom levels to baseline. This may increase the recovery or return to activity time frame significantly.

Tendonitis, particularly in the hip flexor region (iliopsoas, rectus femoris, and tensor fasciae latae) and to a lesser degree the iliotibial band region, has been noted to occur in several individuals postoperatively. Precautions to avoid this complication in individuals undergoing concomitant tissue release procedures are discussed previously. Careful monitoring for symptoms indicative of early development of tendonitis should be exercised. Temporary deferral or modification of aggravating activities is typically the most effective method of addressing this potential complication. Once fully symptomatic, a significant decrease of the majority of activities may be necessary. Various modalities to decrease inflammation and pain may be used, although no strong evidence is available to support the use of specific modalities in this particular population of patients.

The lack of expected progression for ROM is a less common yet an equally as disruptive obstacle that may be encountered during the rehabilitation process. The key factor in treating these occurrences is identification the primary cause. This can be achieved through assessing end-feel, flexibility tests, and mobility testing of the joint. In the middle to later stages of rehabilitation, an empty end-feel associated with significant pain should be a cause of concern. It is generally recommended that patients follow-up with their surgeon for clinical evaluation and diagnostic testing as deemed necessary. When a ROM limitation end-feel is accompanied by a muscular end-feel and clinical tests for decreased flexibility are positive, stretching techniques to improve muscular flexibility are indicated. When the ROM limitation is associated with a more firm/capsular end-feel and tests for joint mobility (manual joint distraction) show decreased motion, manual therapy to increase the mobility characteristics of the joint capsule may be indicated.

OUTCOME: SELF-REPORT INSTRUMENTS

Currently, there is not a universally accepted self-report outcome instrument used to define the result of treatment after hip arthroscopy for FAI. Several instruments are available to specifically assess individuals with musculoskeletal hip pathologies, including, the modified Harris Hip Score and Nonarthritic Hip Score.[12–18] Each of these instruments has potential deficiencies that may have a negative impact on its ability to function as an outcome instrument for individuals with FAI. The Hip Outcome Score

(HOS) is a recently developed instrument with evidence of validity, reliability, and responsiveness to support its use.[19–21] One possible advantage of the HOS is that it contains a separately scored nine-item sports subscale which may be of benefit to those with FAI who are usually functioning at a high level of ability and desire to return to sports.

There is evidence to support the use of the HOS as an outcome instrument for hip arthroscopic hip surgery. This includes evidence for content and construct validity and reliability and responsiveness over a 7-month period for individuals who have undergone arthroscopic hip surgery for FAI.[19–21] Specifically, a score a change beyond 3 points represents a change beyond measurement error for the activities of daily living and sports subscales. An increase in score above 9 and 6 points represents a meaningful increase in score for the activities of daily living and sports subscales respectively.[21] Also, psychometric analysis of the HOS sports subscale has confirmed that it is able to collect information and be potentially responsive for individuals who function at a high level.[19]

OUTCOMES AFTER ARTHROSCOPIC DECOMPRESSION OF FEMOROACETABULAR IMPINGEMENT

Overall, the outcome of hip arthroscopy in adults has been good. It is well documented, however, that the presence of articular cartilage lesions, in particular findings of osteoarthritis, have a negative impact on surgical outcomes.[22–28] Outcome studies for FAI have been reviewed.[1] Open techniques have been historically considered the gold standard for the treatment of FAI. When looking at scientific data for the surgical treatment of labral tears and FAI, however, the seven studies that reported on open techniques did not have better outcomes than the 12 studies that investigated arthroscopic techniques.[22] Outcomes for the arthroscopic technique noted 67% to 100% of patients were satisfied with their outcome.[23,25,29–38] The age for the patients in these 12 studies averaged 33 years (range 29–41 years). Martin and Philippon[21] also reported 2-year outcome data on hip arthroscopy for FAI and associated chondrolabral dysfunction in adults. Overall patient satisfaction was high (median score 9 out 10) with an average improvement of 24 points on modified Harris Hip Score. This study also found those with labral repair had a better outcome than those with labral débridement.[27] When looking specifically at a younger population, a recently study reported short term (1.36 year) outcome information on those with a mean age of 15 years (range 11–16 years).[39] The 16 subjects in this study who were treated for primarily FAI had excellent improvement and a high level of satisfaction. There were no complications associated with slipped capital femoral epiphysis or arrest of the physis.

SUMMARY

The use of arthroscopic technology to address pathologic conditions of the hip joint has become a topic of growing interest in the orthopedic community. Addressing FAI through this method has generated additional attention. As surgical options evolve, rehabilitation protocols must meet the challenge of providing a safe avenue of recovery, yet meeting the goal of returning to often relatively high levels of functioning. Current rehabilitation concepts should be based on the growing body of evidence, knowledge of tissue healing properties, and clinical experience.

REFERENCES

1. Beck M, Kalhor M, Leunig M, et al. Hip morphology influences the pattern of damage to the acetabular cartilage: femoroacetabular impingement as a cause of early osteoarthritis of the hip. J Bone Joint Surg Br 2005;87:1012–8.
2. Ferguson SJ, Bryant JT, Ganz R, et al. An in vitro investigation of the acetabular labral seal in hip joint mechanics. J Biomech 2003;36:171–8.
3. Ferguson SJ, Bryant JT, Ganz R, et al. The influence of the acetabular labrum on hip joint cartilage consolidation: a poroelastic finite element model. J Biomech 2000;33:953–60.
4. Ganz R, Parvizi J, Beck M, et al. Femoroacetabular impingement: a cause for osteoarthritis of the hip. Clin Orthop Relat Res 2003;417:112–20.
5. Ito K, Leunig M, Ganz R. Histopathologic features of the acetabular labrum in femoroacetabular impingement. Clin Orthop Relat Res 2004;429:262–71.
6. Ito K, Minka MA 2nd, Leunig M, et al. Femoroacetabular impingement and the cam-effect. A MRI-based quantitative anatomical study of the femoral head-neck offset. J Bone Joint Surg Br 2001;83:171–6.
7. Leunig M, Beck M, Kalhor M, et al. Fibrocystic changes at anterosuperior femoral neck: prevalence in hips with femoroacetabular impingement. Radiology 2005; 236:237–46.
8. Leunig M, Beck M, Woo A, et al. Acetabular rim degeneration: a constant finding in the aged hip. Clin Orthop Relat Res 2003;413:201–7.
9. Leunig M, Casillas MM, Hamlet M, et al. Slipped capital femoral epiphysis: early mechanical damage to the acetabular cartilage by a prominent femoral metaphysis. Acta Orthop Scand 2000;71:370–5.
10. Enseki KR, Martin R, Draovitch P, et al. The hip joint: arthroscopic procedures and postoperative rehabilitation. J Orthop Sports Phys Ther 2006;36(7):516–25.
11. Garrison JC, Osler MT, Singleton SB. Rehabilitation after arthroscopy of an acetabular labral tear. N Am J Sports Phys Ther 2007;2(4):241–8.
12. Bellamy N, Buchanan WW, Goldsmith CH, et al. Validation study of WOMAC: a health status instrument for measuring clinically important patient relevant outcomes to antirheumatic drug therapy in patients with osteoarthritis of the hip or knee. J Rheumatol 1988;15(12):1833–40.
13. Christensen CP, Althausen PL, Mittleman MA, et al. The nonarthritic hip score: reliable and validated. Clin Orthop Relat Res 2003;406:75–83.
14. Harris WH. Traumatic arthritis of the hip after dislocation and acetabular fractures: treatment by mold arthroplasty. An end-result study using a new method of result evaluation. J Bone Joint Surg Am 1969;51(4):737–55.
15. Hunsaker FG, Cioffi DA, Amadio PC, et al. The American academy of orthopaedic surgeons outcomes instruments: normative values from the general population. J Bone Joint Surg Am 2002;84(2):208–15.
16. Nilsdotter AK, Lohmander LS, Klassbo M, et al. Hip disability and osteoarthritis outcome score (HOOS)–validity and responsiveness in total hip replacement. BMC Musculoskelet Disord 2003;4(1):10.
17. Tugwell P, Bombardier C, Buchanan WW, et al. The MACTAR Patient Preference Disability Questionnaire–an individualized functional priority approach for assessing improvement in physical disability in clinical trials in rheumatoid arthritis. J Rheumatol 1987;14(3):446–51.
18. Wright JG, Young NL, Waddell JP. The reliability and validity of the self-reported patient-specific index for total hip arthroplasty. J Bone Joint Surg Am 2000;82(6): 829–37.

19. Martin RL, Kelly BT, Philippon MJ. Evidence of validity for the hip outcome score. Arthroscopy 2006;22(12):1304–11.
20. Martin RL, Philippon MJ. Evidence of validity for the hip outcome score in hip arthroscopy. Arthroscopy 2007;23(8):822–6.
21. Martin RL, Philippon MJ. Evidence of reliability and responsiveness for the hip outcome score. Arthroscopy 2008;24(6):676–82.
22. Bedi A, Chen N, Robertson W, et al. The management of labral tears and femoroacetabular impingement of the hip in the young, active patient. Arthroscopy 2008;24(10):1135–45.
23. Byrd JW, Jones KS. Prospective analysis of hip arthroscopy with 2-year follow-up. Arthroscopy 2000;16(6):578–87.
24. Byrd JW, Jones KS. Hip arthroscopy for labral pathology: prospective analysis with 10-year follow-up. Arthroscopy 2009;25(4):365–8.
25. Farjo LA, Glick JM, Sampson TG. Hip arthroscopy for acetabular labral tears. Arthroscopy 1999;15(2):132–7.
26. McCarthy JC, Lee J. Hip arthroscopy: indications and technical pearls. Clin Orthop Relat Res 2005;441:180–7.
27. Philippon MJ, Briggs KK, Yen YM, et al. Outcomes following hip arthroscopy for femoroacetabular impingement with associated chondrolabral dysfunction: minimum two-year follow-up. J Bone Joint Surg Br 2009;91(1):16–23.
28. Philippon MJ, Stubbs AJ, Schenker ML, et al. Arthroscopic management of femoroacetabular impingement: osteoplasty technique and literature review. Am J Sports Med 2007;35(9):1571–80.
29. Guanche CA, Sikka RS. Acetabular labral tears with underlying chondromalacia: a possible association with high-level running. Arthroscopy 2005;21(5):580–5.
30. Ilizaliturri VM Jr, Nossa-Barrera JM, Acosta-Rodriguez E, et al. Arthroscopic treatment of femoroacetabular impingement secondary to paediatric hip disorders. J Bone Joint Surg Br 2007;89(8):1025–30.
31. Ilizaliturri VM Jr, Orozco-Rodriguez L, Acosta-Rodriguez E, et al. Arthroscopic treatment of cam-type femoroacetabular impingement: preliminary report at 2 years minimum follow-up. J Arthroplasty 2008;23(2):226–34.
32. Larson CM, Giveans MR. Arthroscopic management of femoroacetabular impingement: early outcomes measures. Arthroscopy 2008;24(5):540–6.
33. McCarthy J, Barsoum W, Puri L, et al. The role of hip arthroscopy in the elite athlete. Clin Orthop Relat Res 2003;406:71–4.
34. O'Leary JA, Berend K, Vail TP. The relationship between diagnosis and outcome in arthroscopy of the hip. Arthroscopy 2001;17(2):181–8.
35. Philippon M, Schenker M, Briggs K, et al. Femoroacetabular impingement in 45 professional athletes: associated pathologies and return to sport following arthroscopic decompression. Knee Surg Sports Traumatol Arthrosc 2007;15(8):1041–7.
36. Potter BK, Freedman BA, Andersen RC, et al. Correlation of Short Form-36 and disability status with outcomes of arthroscopic acetabular labral debridement. Am J Sports Med 2005;33(6):864–70.
37. Santori N, Villar RN. Acetabular labral tears: result of arthroscopic partial limbectomy. Arthroscopy 2000;16(1):11–5.
38. Saw T, Villar R. Footballer's hip a report of six cases. J Bone Joint Surg Br 2004;86(5):655–8.
39. Philippon MJ, Yen YM, Briggs KK, et al. Early outcomes after hip arthroscopy for femoroacetabular impingement in the athletic adolescent patient: a preliminary report. J Pediatr Orthop 2008;28(7):705–10.

Rehabilitation Following Microfracture for Chondral Injury in the Knee

Jason M. Hurst, MD[a], J. Richard Steadman, MD[b], Luke O'Brien, PT[c], William G. Rodkey, DVM, Diplomate ACVS[b], Karen K. Briggs, MPH[b,*]

KEYWORDS

• Microfracture • Chondral injury • Rehabilitation

Full-thickness chondral defects in the knee are common, and these articular cartilage lesions may present in various clinical settings and at different ages.[1–6]

The shearing forces of the femur on the tibia as a single event can result in trauma to the articular cartilage, causing the cartilage to fracture, lacerate, and separate from the underlying subchondral bone or separate with a piece of the subchondral bone.[2,5,6] Chronic repetitive loading in excess of normal physiologic levels may also result in the fatigue and failure of the chondral surface. The single events are usually found in younger groups, whereas chronic degenerative lesions are seen more commonly in the middle-aged and older groups.[2,5–7] It has been shown that repetitive impacts can cause cartilage swelling, an increase in collagen fiber diameter, and an alteration in the relationship between collagen and proteoglycans.[5,6] Acute events, therefore, may not result in full-thickness cartilage loss but rather start a degenerative cascade that can lead to chronic full-thickness loss. The degenerative cascade typically includes early softening and fibrillation (grade I), fissures and cracks in the surface of the cartilage (grade II), severe fissures and cracks with a crab meat appearance (grade III), and, finally, exposure of the subchondral bone (grade IV).[2,5–7]

Articular cartilage defects that extend full thickness to subchondral bone rarely heal without intervention.[1–3,8–19] Some patients may not develop clinically

[a] Joint Implant Surgeons, 7277 Smiths Mill Road, New Albany, OH, USA
[b] Steadman Philippon Research Institute, 181 West Meadow Drive, Suite 1000, Vail, CO 81657, USA
[c] Howard Head Sports Medicine Centers, 181 West Meadow Drive, Vail, CO, USA
* Corresponding author.
E-mail address: Karen.briggs@sprivail.org (K.K. Briggs).

Clin Sports Med 29 (2010) 257–265
doi:10.1016/j.csm.2009.12.009 sportsmed.theclinics.com
0278-5919/10/$ – see front matter

significant problems from acute full-thickness chondral defects, but most eventually suffer from degenerative changes that can be debilitating.[2,3,18–20] Techniques that are used to treat chondral defects include abrasion, drilling, osteochondral autografts, osteochondral allografts, and autologous cell transplantation.[1,2,7,8,20,21] The senior author (JRS) developed the "microfracture" technique to enhance chondral resurfacing by providing a suitable environment for new tissue formation and taking advantage of the body's own healing potential.[8,9,11–17,20–22] The senior author's clinical experience now includes more than 3200 patients who have had the microfracture procedure.

Proper surgical technique is essential, and rehabilitation is equally important. If both are accomplished, the success rate of the microfracture procedure is high. Rehabilitation after microfracture is so important that the microfracture procedure is not performed unless the rehabilitation protocol has been discussed and agreed upon with the patient before surgery. With this combination of surgery and rehabilitation, more invasive procedures, such as osteotomy, cartilage grafting, or unicompartmental arthroplasty, are usually avoided or delayed indefinitely. The goals of this procedure and rehabilitation are to alleviate the pain and disability that can result from chondral lesions and to restore joint conformity, thereby[1,13,20] preventing late degenerative changes in the joint.

POSTOPERATIVE CARE

The postoperative program has been designed to provide the ideal physical environment for the newly recruited mesenchymal stem cells and growth factors from the bone marrow to become a satisfactory cartilage surface.[11,13–15] These differentiation and maturation processes occur slowly and are influenced by the rehabilitation environment.[23,24] Animal studies in horses have confirmed that cellular and molecular changes are an essential part of the development of a durable repair tissue.[21,22]

The authors' experience and clinical research data indicate that improvement can be expected to occur slowly but steadily for at least 2 years.[8,9,11,13,15] During this period, the repair tissue matures, pain and swelling resolve, and the patients regain confidence and comfort in their knees during increased levels of activity.[12]

These factors are critical to designing the ideal postoperative plan.

REHABILITATION PROGRAM

The rehabilitation program after microfracture for the treatment of chondral defects in the knee is crucial to optimize the results of the surgery.[11,23,24] The rehabilitation provides the optimal physical environment for the mesenchymal stem cells to differentiate and produce new cells and extracellular matrix that eventually matures into a durable repair tissue. The surgically induced marrow clot provides the basis for a chemical environment to complement the physical environment.[21,22] This newly proliferated repair cartilage then fills the original defect and matures over time.

The postoperative rehabilitation program after microfracture necessitates consideration of several factors.[11,13,14,23] Because of the variability of chondral defects, including factors such as location and size, the rehabilitation program may need to be altered to accommodate concomitant intra-articular pathology. When other intra-articular procedures, such as anterior cruciate ligament reconstruction, are done concurrently with microfracture, the rehabilitation program is altered as necessary, without interfering with the principles of microfrature healing. The 2 basic protocols that the authors use after microfracture are outlined below.

FEMORAL CONDYLE AND TIBIAL PLATEAU LESIONS

Week 0 to 8

The overall goal of the 0-to-8–week phase post microfracture surgery is to initiate a rehabilitation program that primarily protects the marrow clot, giving a physical message to the new tissue that encourages it to become cartilage, while also restoring full joint range of motion (ROM) and patellar mobility (**Fig. 1**). Additional goals include maintenance of quadriceps function and resolution of joint swelling.

After surgery, patients are placed in a continuous passive motion (CPM) machine set at a range of 30° to 70° and a rate of 1 cycle per minute for 8 hours per day. Superior healing was demonstrated in patients who received CPM as compared with those who did not receive CPM in a postoperative regimen.[9] Most patients are able to tolerate the use of CPM at night. For those who do not, intermittent use during the day is recommended. Patients who cannot tolerate the use of CPM or who cannot obtain reimbursement are instructed to complete 500 flexion/extension ROM exercises 3 times a day.

Protection of the clot created by the microfracture requires that the patient be in touchdown weight bearing for 8 weeks postoperatively (**Fig. 2**). A postoperative brace is rarely used for a lesion of the femoral condyle or tibial plateau. At 8 weeks, the patient is allowed to increase weight bearing to the involved extremity to the point of comfort with the pressure. Upon resuming full weight-bearing status, a compartmental unloader brace may be considered for patients engaging in impact activities, when biomechanical alignment is considered to be a contributing cause of the chondral injury.

Patellar mobilizations are initiated immediately postoperatively and include medial-to-lateral and superior-to-inferior movement of the patella as well as medial-to-lateral movement of the quadriceps and patellar tendon. This mobilization is critical to prevent patellar tendon adhesions (**Fig. 3**) and associated increases in patellofemoral joint reaction forces as previously described by Ahmad and colleagues.[25] Passive flexion and extension (with no ROM limitations) are used day 1 post surgery to restore normal joint ROM. Quadriceps contractions are begun immediately after surgery. Straight leg raises are initiated to restore quadriceps function and muscle control. Cryotherapy is used for all patients in an effort to control pain and swelling.[26] Ankle pumps are encouraged as a prophylaxis for deep vein thrombosis.

Spinning on a stationary bike (no resistance) is initiated 1 to 4 weeks postoperatively. Patients with smaller lesions begin exercises at 1 week, and those with larger

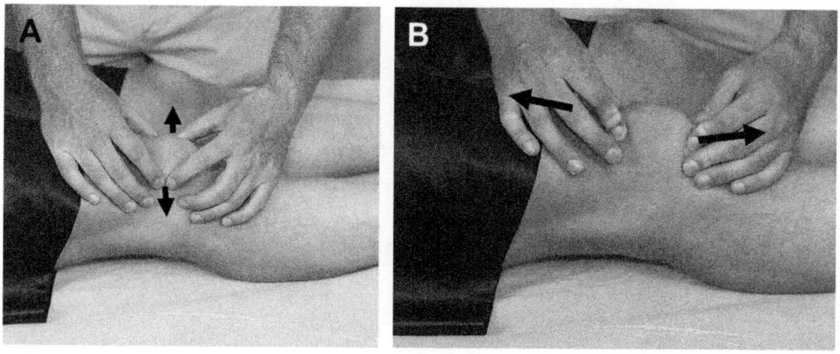

Fig. 1. Patellar mobility exercises are performed (*A*) in the medial-to-lateral direction and (*B*) from the superior to inferior direction.

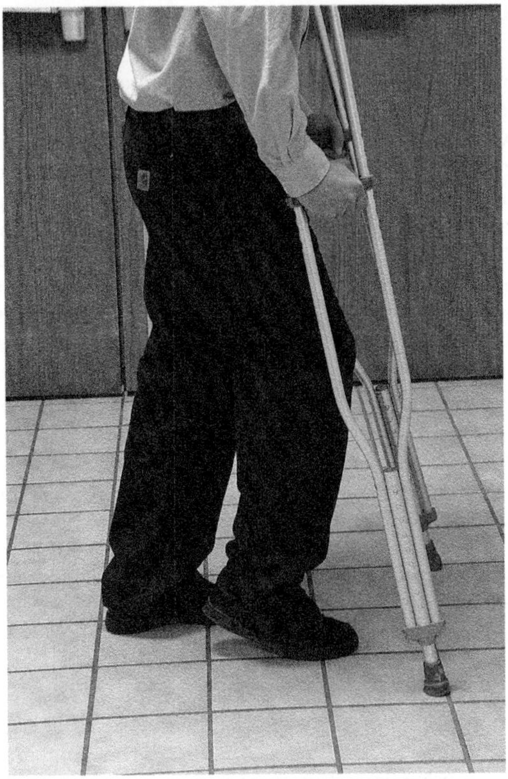

Fig. 2. Touchdown weight bearing is allowed after microfracture.

lesions start at 2 to 4 weeks and progress as tolerated, with a goal of achieving 45 minutes of continuous spinning (5 to 7 days per week) by 8 weeks. Deep water running also begins at 2 weeks unless the lesion is more than 400 mm^2. Patients with larger lesions begin at 4 weeks. It is important that the injured leg does not touch the bottom of the pool during the exercise.

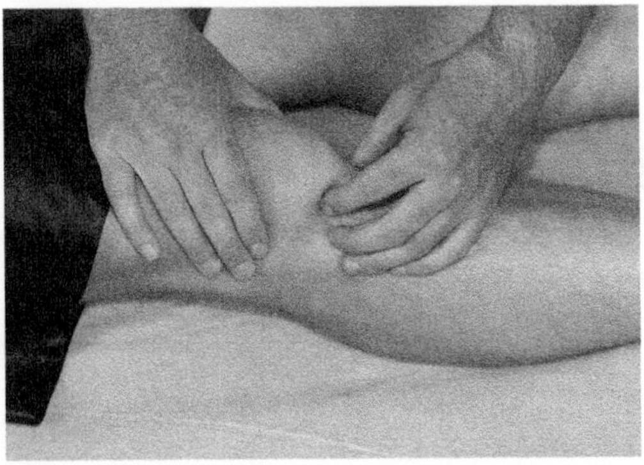

Fig. 3. Mobilization of the patella includes manipulation of the patellar tendon and the quadriceps tendon.

Week 9 to 16

After completion of the initial 8-week healing phase, patients are progressed to weight bearing as tolerated, with most patients weaning off crutches over the period of 1 week.

Once full weight bearing and joint ROM are achieved, the emphasis of the rehabilitation program shifts from a focus on mobility to restoration of normal muscular function. In this phase of rehabilitation, the authors use cardiovascular equipment (stationary bike, treadmill, deep water running, elliptical trainer, and lap kicking in water, with or without kickboard and fins). Closed chain, double-leg exercises with flexion to 30° are allowed. Shallow-range single-leg exercises are allowed at a 0° to 30° range at 3 to 4 months, depending on patient comfort and confidence (**Fig. 4**).

No resistance is used in the stationary bike program until the patient can achieve 45 minutes of pain-free cycling. At this point, tension is gradually increased. The total time is decreased when first adding resistance, to avoid overloading the joint.

Treadmill walking at a 7% incline is introduced at 12 weeks. The impact stress associated with walking dictates that the patient begin with short duration (5–10 minutes) walks with 5-minute progressions added as tolerated. An elliptical trainer may also be used, following the parameters of treadmill walking.

Closed chain exercises are used to build an endurance base on which strength gains can later be made. These exercises are initially double leg, focusing on the major lower extremity muscle groups and using body weight for resistance. Shallow-range single-leg exercises incorporating static holds focus on increasing the ability of the lower extremity muscles to stabilize the knee joint. Therapists should also incorporate exercises that target the stability muscles of the pelvic girdle, because the prolonged period of reduced weight bearing has a deleterious effect on these muscle groups.

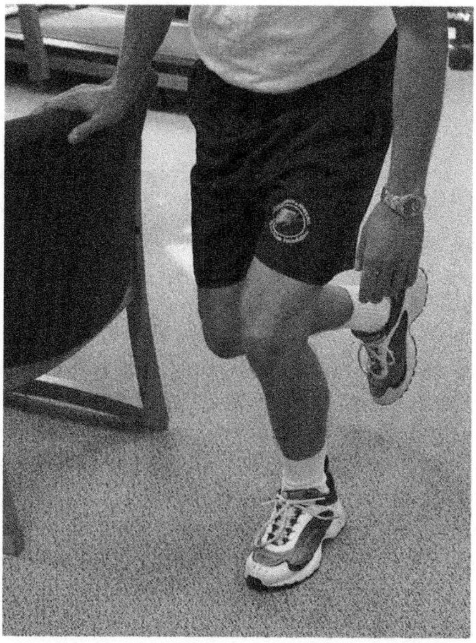

Fig. 4. Single-leg knee bends are allowed but restricted to 30° to 40° at 9 to 16 weeks postoperatively. The timing depends on the lesion and the size of the patient.

Week 17 to 24

With a muscular endurance base built during the 8-to-16–week phase, an emphasis on strength training now predominates. For patients with significant lesions, low-impact exercises, such as those outlined in phase 2, are advanced. For others, progression to single-leg exercise and resistance training is made, with sports specific lifting techniques and strategies implemented when appropriate. Despite full weight-bearing status and pain-free performance of loaded activities, care should still be taken to avoid ranges of motion that affect the microfracture site.

A staged running program may begin at anytime between 16 to 24 weeks, with the determination to start based on the size and severity of the chondral lesion and the patient's sport and recreation. Initial running should take place on a forgiving surface, using 1-minute running followed by 4-minute walking intervals. Running time is increased by 1 minute per week (associated with a 1-minute decrease in walking time) so that the patient is able to complete 20 minutes of continuous running after 5 weeks. Agilities are also initiated once the patient is cleared to commence running. Initial agilities are single-plane activities that are completed at 25% of maximum speed with 25% increases in speed made weekly, and multi-plane activities are added once the running progression is completed.

Week 25 to 36

The final phase of rehabilitation focuses on providing patients with the performance elements that are specific to their sport and recreation. Clearance to return to sport is subject to clinical examination. The authors recommend that patients do not return to sports that involve pivoting, cutting, and jumping until at least 6 to 9 months after microfracture surgery. Persistent effusion, return of localized pain, or loss of motion are signs that the patient is not ready for return to sport and that the patient needs to resume rehabilitation which does not cause these symptoms to occur.

PATELLOFEMORAL LESIONS

All patients are treated with a knee immobilizer set at 0° extension for the first 8 weeks postoperatively. This is done to prevent flexion past the point where the patella engages the trochlear groove, thus minimizing the compressive forces on the microfracture site of the trochlear groove, the patella, or both. After 8 weeks, the brace is opened intermittently before being discontinued.

Patients with patellofemoral lesions are placed in a CPM machine set at 0° to 50° immediately after surgery. Apart from the ROM setting, parameters are the same as those for femorotibial lesions. Although the brace must be worn at all times when the patients are not in the CPM machine, they are allowed to bear partial weight (30% body weight) immediately postoperatively, with progression to weight bearing as tolerated after 2 weeks. In larger lesions (more than 400 mm^2), weight bearing is protected for 4 to 6 weeks. Typically, patients are allowed full passive ROM immediately after surgery. The presence of kissing lesions, multiple defects, or defects of significant size, however, may limit ROM parameters.

During completion of the microfracture procedure, particular notice is paid to the femorotibial angle at which the patellofemoral-chondral defect is engaged. During strength training, these angles should be avoided for approximately 4 to 6 months. Apart from this angle avoidance, the strengthening exercise program is the same as that used for femorotibial lesions.

Joint environment affects the healing time of defects. For example, patients with previous meniscectomies have less protection for the maturing cartilage. In these and similar cases, the total rehabilitation time is increased by 2 to 3 months.

CLINICAL RESULTS OF MICROFRACTURE

The first long-term outcomes report on the microfracture technique was published in 2003.[11] This study followed up 72 patients younger than 45 years for an average of 11 years after microfracture (range, 7 to 17 years). This study was limited to knees with no joint space narrowing, no degenerative arthritis, and no ligament or meniscus pathology that required treatment. With a 95% follow-up rate, the results showed improvement in symptoms and function. Patients reported that pain and swelling were decreased at postoperative year 1, continued to decrease at year 2, and the clinical improvements were maintained during the study period. The study identified age as the only independent predictor of Lysholm improvement. Patients older than 35 years improved less than patients who were younger; however, both groups showed improvement.[11]

Cartilage injuries are common in high-impact sports. The authors documented the outcome of microfracture in patients who played professional football in the United States.[27] Twenty-five active National Football League players were treated with microfracture between 1986 and 1997. The study found that 76% of players returned to play the next football season. After return to play, those same players played an average of 4.6 additional seasons. All players showed decreased symptoms and improvement in function. Of those players who did not return to play, most had preexisting degenerative changes of the knee.[27]

The important common factors between these 2 studies and other similar reports on microfracture from the authors' institution are (1) strict adherence to the described rehabilitation protocol, (2) careful patient selection, and (3) resisting the temptation to advance patients too rapidly through the prescribed therapy regimen. Early weight bearing or premature return to shear-producing joint forces will likely compromise the clinical benefits of microfracture and potentially create a lesion that is less receptive to joint preservation.

SUMMARY

Based on the authors' extensive clinical experience, it may be concluded that arthroscopic debridement and microfracture of subchondral bone is safe and effective to treat full-thickness chondral defects of the knee. Microfracture in combination with the appropriate rehabilitation protocol significantly improves functional outcomes and decreases pain in most patients who are treated.

REFERENCES

1. Brittberg M, Lindahl A, Nilsson A, et al. Treatment of deep cartilage defects in the knee with autologous chondrocyte transplantation. N Engl J Med 1994;331:889–95.
2. Blevins FT, Steadman JR, Rodrigo JJ, et al. Treatment of articular cartilage defects in athletes: an analysis of functional outcome and lesion appearance. Orthopedics 1998;21:761–8.
3. Cohen NP, Foster RJ, Mow VC. Composition and dynamics of articular cartilage: structure, function, and maintaining healthy state. J Orthop Sports Phys Ther 1998;28:203–15.

4. DePalma AF, McKeever CD, Subin DK. Process of repair of articular cartilage demonstrated by histology and autoradiography with tritiated thymidine. Clin Orthop 1966;48:229–42.
5. Mankin HJ. Reaction of articular cartilage to injury and osteoarthritis. N Engl J Med 1974;291:1335–40.
6. Mankin HJ. The response of articular cartilage to mechanical injury. J Bone Joint Surg Am 1982;64:460–5.
7. Johnson LL. The sclerotic lesion: pathology and the clinical response to arthroscopic abrasion arthroplasty. In: Ewing JW, editor. Articular cartilage and knee joint function: basic science and arthroscopy. New York: Raven Press; 1990. p. 319–33.
8. Buckwalter JA. Articular cartilage: injuries and potential for healing. J Orthop Sports Phys Ther 1998;28:192–202.
9. Rodrigo JJ, Steadman JR, Silliman JF, et al. Improvement of full-thickness chondral defect healing in the human knee after debridement and microfracture using continuous passive motion. Am J Knee Surg 1994;7:109–16.
10. Singleton SB, Silliman JF. Acute chondral injuries of the patellofemoral joint. Oper Tech Sports Med 1995;3:96–103.
11. Steadman JR, Briggs KK, Rodrigo JJ, et al. Outcomes of microfracture for traumatic chondral defects of the knee: average 11-year follow-up. Arthroscopy 2003;19:477–84.
12. Steadman JR, Rodkey WG. Microfracture in the pediatric and adolescent knee. In: Micheli LJ, Kocher M, editors. The pediatric and adolescent knee. Philadelphia: WB Saunders; 2006.
13. Steadman JR, Rodkey WG, Briggs KK. Microfracture chondroplasty: indications, techniques, and outcomes. Sports Med Arthrosc Rev 2003;11:236–44.
14. Steadman JR, Rodkey WG, Briggs KK. Microfracture to treat full-thickness chondral defects. J Knee Surg 2002;15:170–6.
15. Steadman JR, Rodkey WG, Rodrigo JJ. Microfracture: surgical technique and rehabilitation to treat chondral defects. Clin Orthop Relat Res 2001;391(Suppl): S362–9.
16. Steadman JR, Rodkey WG, Singleton SB, et al. Microfracture procedure for treatment of full-thickness chondral defects: technique, clinical results and current basic science status. In: Harner CD, Vince KG, Fu FH, editors. Techniques in knee surgery. Media. Philadelphia: Williams & Wilkins; 1999. p. 23–31.
17. Steadman JR, Rodkey WG, Singleton SB, et al. Microfracture technique for full-thickness chondral defects: technique and clinical results. Oper Tech Orthop 1997;7:300–4.
18. Urrea LH, Silliman JF. Acute chondral injuries to the femoral condyles. Oper Tech Sports Med 1995;3:104–11.
19. Walker JM. Pathomechanics and classification of cartilage lesions, facilitation of repair. J Orthop Sports Phys Ther 1998;28:216–31.
20. Steadman JR, Rodkey WG, Briggs KK, et al. Debridement and microfracture for full-thickness articular cartilage defects. In: Scott WN, editor. Insall and Scott surgery of the knee. Philadelphia: Churchill Livingstone Elsevier; 2006. p. 359–66.
21. Frisbie DD, Oxford JT, Southwood L, et al. Early events in cartilage repair after subchondralbone microfracture. Clin Orthop 2003;407:215–27.
22. Frisbie DD, Trotter GW, Powers BE, et al. Arthroscopic subchondral bone plate microfracture technique augments healing of large osteochondral defects in the radial carpal bone and medial femoral condyle of horses. Vet Surg 1999; 28:242–55.

23. Hagerman GR, Atkins JA, Dillman C. Rehabilitation of chondral injuries and chronic degenerative arthritis of the knee in the athlete. Oper Tech Sports Med 1995;3:127–35.
24. Irrgang JJ, Pezzullo D. Rehabilitation following surgical procedures to address articular cartilage lesions of the knee. J Orthop Sports Phys Ther 1998;28: 232–40.
25. Ahmad CS, Kwak SD, Ateshian GA, et al. Effects of patellar tendon adhesion to the anterior tibia on knee mechanics. Am J Sports Med 1998;26:715–24.
26. Ohkoshi Y, Ohkoshi M, Nagasaki S, et al. The effect of cryotherapy on intraarticular temperature and postoperative care after anterior cruciate ligament reconstruction. Am J Sports Med 1999;27:357–62.
27. Steadman JR, Miller BS, Karas SG, et al. The microfracture technique in the treatment of full-thickness chondral lesions of the knee in National Football League players. J Knee Surg 2003;16:83–6.

Rehabilitation After Autologous Chondrocyte Implantation in Athletes

Shane J. Nho, MD, MS[a,*], Michael J. Pensak, MD[b], Daniel A. Seigerman, MD[c], Brian J. Cole, MD, MBA[a]

KEYWORDS

- Autologous chondrocyte implantation • Rehabilitation
- Wound healing • Plyometrics

Articular cartilage is a vital joint structure as evidenced by the progressive, painful, and debilitating loss of joint function that occurs when it becomes damaged. The importance of articular cartilage is evident in large, weight-bearing joints of the body, particularly the hip, knee, shoulder, and ankle, which are subjected to tremendous shear, tensile, and compressive forces with daily activities. Athletes may also sustain focal chondral injuries after an acute traumatic event, or insidiously, secondary to repetitive overuse due to the abnormal joint demands. Over the years a variety of cartilage restorative procedures have been developed to address focal, full-thickness cartilaginous defects in the knee joint, including microfracture, osteochondral autografts, osteochondral allografts, autologous chondrocyte implantation (ACI), and most recently, next-generation ACI involving scaffolds or cell-seeded scaffolds. Since its introduction, ACI has yielded some very promising results in athletes and nonathletes alike. Rehabilitation following ACI requires an in-depth understanding of joint mechanics, and knowledge of the biologic and biomechanical properties of healing articular cartilage. A patient-, lesion-, and sports-specific approach is required on the part of the trainer or physical therapist to gradually restore knee joint function and strength so that the athlete may be able to return to competitive play.

[a] Cartilage Restoration Center, Division of Sports Medicine, Department of Orthopedic Surgery, Midwest Orthopaedics at Rush, Rush University Medical Center, Rush Medical College of Rush University, 1725 West Harrison Street, Suite 1063, Chicago, IL 60607, USA
[b] Department of Orthopaedic Surgery, University of Connecticut, 263 Farmington Avenue, Medical Arts Building, Farmington, CT 06030, USA
[c] Department of Orthopaedic Surgery, New Jersey Medical School, University of Medicine and Dentistry of New Jersey, 90 Bergen Street, Newark, NJ 07101, USA
* Corresponding author.
E-mail address: sjaynho@rushortho.com (S.J. Nho).

Clin Sports Med 29 (2010) 267–282
doi:10.1016/j.csm.2009.12.004
sportsmed.theclinics.com
0278-5919/10/$ – see front matter

ATHLETES TREATED WITH ACI

Cartilaginous defects are typically caused by repetitive shear forces, torsional loads, or high-impact stress.[1] The prevalence of these lesions in the general public is difficult to determine but estimates suggest that approximately 5% of the population have a focal, full-thickness cartilaginous defect.[1] Among patients undergoing knee arthroscopy, the prevalence of full-thickness defects is much higher. One series of 31,516 knee arthroscopies noted a 63% prevalence of chondral lesions, with 19.2% having grade IV chondromalacia.[2]

The prevalence of articular cartilage abnormalities in a general athletic population is not known but is thought to be much higher than the general population. There are sports-specific articular cartilage injury patterns depending on the type of physical demands on the knee. In a study by Walczak and colleagues,[3] 14 male National Basketball Association (NBA) players obtained bilateral knee magnetic resonance imaging (MRI) before the start of the season to evaluate for abnormalities in asymptomatic players with MRI. The investigators determined that 25 of 28 (89.3%) knees had abnormalities on routine preseason MRI for asymptomatic knees. Fifty percent of the players had an abnormal signal in the articular cartilage, which was consistent with the findings of 2 other studies that reported the prevalence of abnormal articular cartilage in 41% of collegiate basketball and 47.5% of NBA players.[4,5] The incidence of cartilaginous joint abnormalities in the general population was estimated at 3.7% in another study.[6] Eckstein and colleagues[7] conducted studies using MRI and 3-dimensional digital image analysis to determine the amount of cartilage deformation with certain activities. These investigators determined that cartilage deformation was significantly higher in the patellofemoral joint than the tibiofemoral joint.[7] Given the amount of jumping and direct knee contact in basketball players, it is not surprising that there is such a high prevalence of patellofemoral joint articular cartilage injuries. Mithofer and colleagues[8] reported that in high-level soccer players 48% of cartilage defects occurred on the medial femoral condyle, 23% occurred on the lateral femoral condyle, and only 29% occurred in the patellofemoral joint. Although the clinical examination is critical when evaluating an in-season injury, the investigators advocate that a preseason MRI for professional athletes is extremely helpful in providing information on interval change in the setting of a new injury and providing prognostic information related to decisions regarding return to play.[3]

There are certain patient- and lesion-specific factors associated with an improvement in knee functional outcomes as well as the ability to return to play.[8,9] For example, younger patient age has been associated with more favorable outcomes in several studies.[8–12] Cartilage injuries in competitive adolescent or young adult athletes may occur after an acute traumatic injury or injury to the cartilage secondary to osteochondritis dissecans (OCD).[9] In skeletally immature patients, these injuries generally result from a shearing force through the zone of provisional calcification of the open physis, which is structurally similar to the articular cartilage.[9] Acute treatment with either repair or replacement results in a higher potential for healing in younger patients.[13] However, Mithofer and colleagues[8] reported that there was no statistically significant difference between the clinical outcomes scores or return to play in a cohort of 20 soccer players treated with ACI in terms of the status of the physis or the mechanism of injury (an acute traumatic episode or OCD).[8,14] The investigators also determined that the mean age of patients that returned to sport was 22.3 years versus 27.6 years in patients who did not return to sport, and there was also a higher proportion of high-level athletes among patients who returned to sport.[8] There are several reasons for improved outcomes in high-level athletes, including acuity of injury, younger age, improved rehabilitation, and higher motivation.[8,15]

The duration of symptoms has been reported by several studies to affect the functional outcome.[8,16] ACI performed within 1 year after injury has a much higher likelihood of a return to preinjury level of sports compared with those that are treated after a prolonged period of symptoms. Although there are no definitive reasons for lower rate of return, chronic cartilage lesions may increase in size, affect the opposite articular surface, and contribute to an unfavorable repair environment. The delay in treatment also affects the ability to return to preinjury levels of sports due to deconditioning or relative inactivity.[8,17] Several studies have demonstrated that the number of prior procedures may also affect the overall functional outcome and return to preinjury athletics.[8,18,19]

Lesion characteristics also affect the overall knee function. Larger lesions have been reported to have less favorable results as well as knees with more than one cartilage lesion.[8,18,20,21] Medial femoral condyle articular cartilage injures also have been shown to have improved outcomes over other areas of the knee. Concomitant abnormalities including malalignment, meniscal deficiency, and ligamentous instability increase the complexity of the operative intervention but also improve the clinical outcomes in patients undergoing cartilage repair. For example, in one study there was no significant difference between soccer players who underwent isolated ACI and those who underwent ACI with osteotomy, meniscus repair, or anterior cruciate ligament reconstruction in terms of return to play.[8] In fact, failure to recognize and treat combined pathology may result in repeat surgical intervention and prolonged rehabilitation. The results of ACI in general are well reported in the literature, and support good to excellent outcomes in both the patellofemoral and tibiofemoral joint.[22–24]

BIOLOGY OF ACI HEALING

The rationale behind the development of ACI for the treatment of full-thickness chondral injuries is based on the unique biology of articular cartilage. In well-vascularized tissue, inflammatory mediators are recruited to aid in the healing process. However, articular cartilage has poor vascular supply, hindering its ability to repair cartilage damage.[1,25,26] Despite early research in the 1980s by Grande and colleagues[27] that highlighted the ability of chondrocytes to replicate when isolated enzymatically from their matrix, in vivo they have a very limited capacity to migrate to sites of injury.[28] Left alone, full-thickness articular cartilage defects will, at best, not heal, and more likely continue to enlarge by circumferential expansion, exposing increasing amounts of subchondral bone, potentially predisposing the knee to accelerated arthrosis. Because the average depth of articular cartilage on the femur, patella, and knee are only 2.0, 3.33, and 2.92 mm, respectively, even partial-thickness lesions may progress to exposed subchondral bone with even minor degrees of defect progression.[29]

Of critical importance in the rehabilitation process following ACI is graft incorporation, maturation, and production of extracellular matrix. Understanding the timeline for tissue maturation helps to guide the principles of postoperative rehabilitation such that tissue development is promoted while simultaneously preventing mechanical overload from occurring. A significant advantage of ACI over other procedures that aim to fill contained articular cartilage defects is the formation of predominantly hyaline or hyalinelike cartilage.[30] Although the ultimate goal of cartilage transplantation procedures is to restore the structure of native cartilage on both a microscopic and macroscopic level, the process is not instantaneous and requires a complex, temporal cascade of cellular division and incorporation into host tissue. Whereas the specific details of this intricate cascade are generally unknown, various studies have looked at the histology of graft tissue at various periods after implantation.

Canine studies have been instrumental in highlighting the various stages of chondrocyte healing.[31] The first 6 weeks constitute the proliferative phase of healing whereby a primitive cellular response leads to tissue fill of the defect. Grande and colleagues[27] demonstrated that within 6 weeks of implantation, autologous chondrocytes underwent significant division and became incorporated into reconstituted cartilage matrix. Their work solidified the idea that the transplanted cells survive and divide after transplantation, and do not merely act to induce articular growth from within the host's intact cartilage matrix. A transition phase, lasting from 3 to 6 months, follows the proliferative response. During this crucial period proteoglycan production occurs, although it is still poorly integrated and takes on a more fluid consistency. At the 6-month time point the graft is usually firm and has incorporated into adjacent articular cartilage and subchondral bone, which typically correlates with a reduction in a patient's symptoms. Remodeling and maturation take place on larger time scales, between 2 and 3 years following ACI. The seminal events during this period include the formation of cross-links between matrix proteins and aggregate formation leading to improved stability and integration into subchondral bone. Throughout all these stages of graft healing a fine balance must be maintained to promote matrix synthesis and graft incorporation without exposing the chondrocytes to excessive loads.[31]

In a translational project by Brittberg and colleagues,[32] the group demonstrated histologic changes over time in the rabbit patellae. At 8 and 12 weeks following ACI, the implanted chondrocytes demonstrated rich cluster formation indicating mitotic activity. Exactly 1 year following ACI, the histologic characteristics of the repaired cartilage appeared more columnar in nature and showed signs of integration with the adjacent, healthy cartilage.

REHABILITATION PROTOCOL

The rehabilitation protocol is critical for successful recovery from ACI surgery and return to high-demand athletic activity. It is generally accepted that the 3 phases of the maturation process for ACI rehabilitation are proliferative, matrix production, and maturation phases.[33,34] The proliferative phase occurs soon after implantation of the autologous chondrocytes, followed by matrix production in which the tissue becomes incorporated into the surrounding host cartilage.[35] In the recovery phase, the ACI continues to mature and the biomechanical properties begin to resemble the surrounding articular cartilage. These goals are achieved by a combination of progressive weight bearing, restoration of range of motion, improving muscle control and strengthening, and sport-specific activities.

Phase 1: Femoral Condyles

Many studies have shown the importance of joint motion after cartilage implantation. Continuous passive motion (CPM) postoperatively, as well as weight-bearing activities, are associated with proteoglycan and collagen reorganization.[36,37] Weight-bearing activity is typically withheld until after the first 2 weeks of implantation to preserve physical properties of the graft. In subsequent studies looking at long-term outcomes for ACI, histologic analysis demonstrated that biopsies from weight-bearing surfaces appeared to resemble organized hyaline cartilage with type II collagen. Biopsies in nonweight-bearing areas resembled fibrocartilage.[25] Peterson and colleagues[25] reported that the biopsied samples demonstrating a hyalinelike cartilaginous content do, in fact, have a superficial fibrous layer indicating periosteal remnant. This finding did not affect the clinical success of the graft.

Traditional thinking asserts that a graduated program of weight bearing and controlled exercise will provide a healthy intra-articular environment for the graft.[38,39] Such protocols recommend an initial 2 weeks of nonweight bearing (NWB) followed by partial weight bearing (PWB) up until 4 weeks after surgery (**Tables 1** and **2**). From 4 to 6 weeks, the patient may progress to the use of one crutch, with gradual increases in load over the following 6 weeks so that full weight bearing (FWB) occurs by week 12.[40] Investigators working with second- and third-generation ACI techniques employing collagen scaffolds (CACI) and matrix-induced ACI (MACI), respectively, recently have advocated more aggressive rehabilitation regimens. Robertson and colleagues[38] still advocate obtaining FWB by the twelfth postoperative week. However, rather than having an initial 6 weeks of toe-touch ambulation only, they believe patients should gradually progress from 20% of their body weight (BW) at 2 weeks after the operation through to FWB at 12 weeks. In a randomized controlled trial of patients undergoing MACI, Ebert and colleagues[41] found that compared with a standard rehabilitation regimen, patients in the accelerated rehabilitation group (FWB achieved by eighth postoperative week) had reduced knee pain, improved function, and greater 6-minute walk distances and daily activity levels. However, because MACI is often performed in a less invasive fashion and is performed without periosteal sutures compared with first-generation ACI, such accelerated protocols may not be applicable to conventional ACI.[42] The authors' current approach, especially for contained lesions, involves initial heel-touch or toe-touch weight bearing, as this has not been shown to be detrimental to graft integration and facilitates transition activities (ie, arising from a bed or chair to a standing position), which are very difficult for patients to perform when completely NWB. In addition, the authors use a brace that has off-loading capability (TROM Adjuster; Don Joy Orthopedics, Carlsbad, CA, USA), which incorporates the same 3-point bending principles as a brace typically prescribed for osteoarthritis. As weight bearing is advanced, the maximal amount of off-loading that the patient can tolerate to facilitate relative unicompartmental unloading is "dialed in" while the patient is simultaneously reactivating frontal and posterior chain musculature.

A knowledge of joint kinematics, taking into account the areas of contact, loads, and pressures generated during normal joint movements, is essential for designing rational rehabilitation protocols that minimize damage to the graft and promote healing (see **Tables 1** and **2**). The tibiofemoral joint (TFJ), a modified hinge joint, possesses 6 degrees of freedom that result in a combination of rolling and gliding as the knee moves through flexion to extension.[43,44] Safe rehabilitation protocols must minimize shear and compressive forces on the articular cartilage. For the initial 2 weeks, the patient is placed in a locked, hinged knee brace in extension for ambulation, but this may be removed for CPM and exercise. Over the next 2 weeks, the brace can be gradually opened 20° at a time as quadriceps control is regained, and the brace may be discontinued when the quadriceps is able to control a straight leg raise without an extension lag. CPM is used for the first 4 weeks for 6 to 8 hours per day at 1 cycle per minute, beginning at 0° to 30° increasing roughly 5° to 10° daily, with the goal of 90° by week 4 and 120° to 130° by week 6. Therapeutic exercise begins with attempting to restore quadriceps control with quad sets, straight leg raises, and hamstring isometrics for the first 2 weeks. Closed chain exercises are initiated between 2 and 6 weeks after surgery, with progressive strengthening over the course of the first 3 months. Again, knowledge of defect location is necessary, because during many activities only certain aspects of the TFJ are in contact.[43,45] If the ACI site is located in the anterior aspect of the joint, full extension with closed chain activities is to be

Table 1
Autologous chondrocyte implantation (femoral condyle only) rehabilitation protocol

	Weight Bearing	Brace	Rom	Therapeutic Exercise
PHASE 1 (0–12 weeks)	**0–2 weeks**: Nonweight bearing **2–4 weeks**: Partial weight bearing (30–40 lbs) **4–6 weeks**: Progress to use of one crutch **6–12 weeks**: Progress to full weight bearing	**0–2 weeks**: Locked in full extension (removed for CPM and exercise) **2–4 weeks**: Gradually open brace 20° at a time as quad control is gained; discontinue use of brace when quads can control straight leg raises without an extension lag	**0–4 weeks:** CPM: use in 2-h increments for 6–8 h per day at 1 cycle/min—begin at 0°–30° increasing 5°–10° daily per patient comfort; patient should gain at least 90° by week 4 and 120°–130° by week 6	**0–2 weeks**: Quad sets, straight leg raises, hamstring isometrics; complete exercises in brace if quad control is inadequate **2–6 weeks**: Begin progressive closed chain exercises[a] **6–10 weeks**: Progress bilateral closed chain strengthening, begin opened chain knee strengthening **10–12 weeks**: Progress closed chain exercises using resistance less than patient's body weight, progress to unilateral closed chain exercises, begin balance activities
PHASE 2 (12 weeks to 6 months)	Full with a normalized gait pattern	None	Full active range of motion	Advance bilateral and unilateral closed chain exercises with emphasis on concentric/eccentric control, continue with biking, stairmaster and treadmill, progress balance activities

PHASE 3 (6–9 months)	Full with a normalized gait pattern	None	Full and pain free	Advance strength training, initiate light plyometrics and jogging—start with 2-min walk/2-min jog, emphasize sport-specific training
PHASE 4 (9–18 months)	Full with a normalized gait pattern	None	Full and pain free	Continue strength training—emphasize single leg loading, begin a progressive running and agility program; high-impact activities (basketball, tennis, etc) may begin at 16 months if pain free

[a] Respect chondrocyte graft site with closed chain activities: if anterior, avoid loading in full extension; if posterior, avoid loading in flexion >45°.
[b] If pain or swelling occurs with any activities, they must be modified to decrease symptoms.

Table 2
Autologous chondrocyte implantation (trochlea/patella)[a] rehabilitation protocol

	Weight Bearing	Brace	Rom	Therapeutic Exercise
PHASE 1 (0–12 weeks)	**0–2 weeks**: Nonweight bearing **2–4 weeks**: Partial weight bearing (30–40 lbs) **4–8 weeks**: Continue with partial weight-bearing status, progress to use of one crutch **8–12 weeks**: Progress to full weight bearing and discard crutches	**0–2 weeks**: Locked in full extension (removed for CPM and exercise) **2–4 weeks**: Locked at 0° with weight bearing **4–6 weeks**: Begin to open 20°–30° with ambulation; discontinue use after 6 weeks	**0–4 weeks**: CPM: use in 2-h increments for 6–8 h per day at 1 cycle/min—begin at 0°–30°; after week 3, increase flexion by 5°–10° daily **6–8 weeks**: Gain 0°–90° **8 weeks**: Gain 0°–120°	**1–4 weeks**: Quad sets, straight leg raises, hamstring isometrics—complete exercises in brace if quad control is inadequate **4–10 weeks**: Begin *isometric* closed chain exercises; at 6–10 weeks, may begin weight shifting activities with involved leg extended if full weight bearing; at 8 weeks begin balance activities and stationary bike with light resistance **10–12 weeks**: Hamstring strengthening, theraband 0°–30° resistance, light open chain knee isometrics
PHASE 2 (12 weeks to 6 months)	Full with a normalized gait pattern	None	Full range of motion	Begin treadmill walking at a slow to moderate pace, progress balance/proprioceptive activities, initiate sport cord lateral drills

PHASE 3 (6–9 months)	Full with a normalized gait pattern	None	Full and pain free	Advance closed chain strengthening, initiate unilateral closed chain exercises, progress to fast walking and backward walking on treadmill (initiate incline at 8–10 months), initiate light plyometric activity
PHASE 4 (9–18 months)	Full with a normalized gait pattern	None	Full and pain free	Continue strength training—emphasize single leg loading, begin a progressive running and agility program; high-impact activities may begin at 16 months

Note: Postoperative stiffness in flexion following trochlear/patellar implantation is not uncommon, and patients are encouraged to achieve 90° of flexion at least 3 times/day out of the brace after their first postoperative visit (days 7–10).

[a] Most trochlear/patellar defect repairs are performed in combination with a distal realignment procedure.

[b] May consider patellofemoral taping or stabilizing brace if improper patella tracking stresses implantation.

[c] If pain or swelling occurs with any activities, they must be modified to decrease symptoms.

avoided. If the ACI site is posterior, loading in flexion greater than 45° with closed chain activities should be avoided.

Phase 1: Patellofemoral

The patellofemoral joint (PFJ) is designed to increase the mechanical advantage of the quadriceps mechanism while minimizing focal cartilage stresses by distributing force equally to the underlying bone. The patella has the thickest articular cartilage in the human body as well as a broad articulating surface.[46–48] At full, passive extension the patella rests on the supratrochlear fat pad, avoiding any contact with the femoral articular surface. Up to a certain point, increasing knee flexion results in concomitant increases in the patellofemoral joint reaction force (PFJRF) and contact areas. Initial contact between the patella and femur occurs at 10 degrees of flexion as the inferior pole of the patella engages the trochlea. At 60 degrees of flexion, the middle surface of patella makes contact with the middle third of the trochlea. Over these 50 degrees, mean contact area increases from 126 to 560 mm^3.[35,49] Optimizing the PFJ contact area as opposed to decreasing the force promotes better nutrient exchange of the cartilage and decreases the pressure on the PFJ.[44,48,50,51]

Patellofemoral ACI is typically performed with tibial tubercle anteromedialization (AMZ), and the first phase of rehabilitation is slower than ACI of the femoral condyles.[22] Weight-bearing activity is typically limited to heel- or toe-touch weight bearing until after the 3 to 4 weeks of implantation, when an AMZ is performed to prevent a postoperative tibial shaft insufficiency fracture. When no AMZ is performed, the authors liberally advance to weight bearing as tolerated with crutches while locked in extension, as patellofemoral forces are not altered significantly with WB when in extension. A locked, hinged knee brace is used for the first 4 weeks and is removed for CPM or exercise. At 4 weeks, the hinged knee brace may be opened 20° to 30° with ambulation and may be discontinued after 6 weeks. CPM is initiated immediately after surgery for 6 to 8 hours per day beginning from 0° to 30° at 1 cycle per minute. After 3 weeks, the flexion may be increased to 5° to 10° daily with the goal of 90° by 6 to 8 weeks and 0° to 120° by 8 weeks after surgery. Because of their initial experience following patellofemoral ACI whereby there was a small incidence of difficulties in regaining full flexion, the authors encourage patients to achieve up to 90 degrees of flexion by simply dangling the foot while sitting in a chair for up to 3 times per day beginning at postoperative week 2.

Therapeutic exercise begins with attempting to restore quadriceps control with quad sets, straight leg raises, and hamstring isometrics for the first 4 weeks. Isometric closed chain exercises are initiated between 6 and 10 weeks after surgery, and patients may begin weight-shifting activities in extension. If FWB by 8 weeks, the patient may begin balance activities with light resistance on a stationary bicycle. The patient may continue progressive strengthening over the course of the first 3 months with the use of a theraband and light open chain knee isometrics.

Phase 2

By 3 months after surgery, the patient has recovered full active range of motion with a normalized gait pattern. Patients who have undergone ACI of the femoral condyles may continue to advance with closed chain activities with an emphasis on concentric/eccentric control. A stationary bicycle can be introduced early in the rehabilitation process, but it is important to use minimal resistance in the beginning to allow complete pedal revolution. The saddle height has a direct influence on knee flexion angles and needs to be appropriate for the specific ACI graft location.[52] For example, the lower the saddle height, the higher the patellofemoral joint reactive force; and the higher the saddle height, the lower the range of knee flexion.[39,53] Saddle height can be raised initially to allow a complete pedal revolution and restrict excessive knee flexion, but the seat should be lowered to the appropriate height as range of motion is restored. Other low-impact exercise modalities with a stair stepper, elliptical trainer, or treadmill can also be considered, but there is a lack of clinical and biomechanical data available.[39]

Patients who have undergone ACI of the patellofemoral joint may begin treadmill walking at a slow pace and may progress to a moderate pace. Neuromuscular re-education and proprioceptive activities are critical components for patellofemoral ACI rehabilitation. Patellofemoral pain syndrome has been reported to be associated with proprioceptive deficits.[54] The relationship between articular cartilage lesions and proprioception is not known; however, open procedures are thought to result in increased proprioceptive loss due to increased disruption of joint mechanoreceptors.[55,56] ACI rehabilitation should focus on restoring proprioception in a dynamic, functional manner with an emphasis on neuromuscular control to retrain coordination patterns.[39] In the early stages, patients are encouraged to vary movement speeds to target the feedback systems and progress to faster movements that focus on retraining the feed-forward system.[39] There are several exercises that can be performed, including eyes open to shut, 2-legged to 1-legged stance, unstable base, resistance or center of gravity shift, and sports-specific drills.[39]

Phase 3

At 6 to 9 months after surgery, the patient should continue the progressive strength training and transition to more functional activities. Patients should continue closed chain strengthening with a treadmill, beginning with a slow walking pace and eventually to a light jog over the course of the next 3 months. Patellofemoral patients should also incorporate backward walking on a treadmill at the 8- to 10-month time point. During this phase, athletes should also begin a core strengthening program and initiate plyometric activity.

Core stability is an important component of any lower extremity rehabilitation program and also has a role in postoperative ACI rehabilitation. A recent prospective study by Leetun and colleagues[57] measured the femoral abduction and external rotation isometric force as well as abdominal, back extension, and quadratus lumborum endurance in preseason intercollegiate athletes. Those athletes with weaker preseason femoral abduction and external strength were more likely to sustain an in-season injury.[57] Additional studies also support the participation of a neuromuscular training program for lower extremity injury prevention.[34,52]

Core strengthening should focus on isometric cocontractions of the lumbar multifidus and transversus abdominis during functional activities.[58] Patients should maintain a neutral spinal position and gently draw in the abdominal wall by contracting the lumbar multifidus.[59] The patient should begin to perform drawing-in exercises in positions of greater support and progress to functional positions while dissociating extremity movements. Specific core muscle strengthening exercises can be done with curl-ups or side planks. Equipment involving exercise balls, foam rollers, platforms, and balance boards can be implemented to increase external torque for further core strengthening. Strengthening of the hip abductors and external rotators are critical to maintain proper lower extremity alignment and prevention of potential knee injuries. The rationale behind a plyometric program is to train the muscles, connective tissue, and nervous system to carry out stretch-shortening cycle focusing of proper technique and mechanics.[60] A recent systematic review concluded that plyometrics, dynamic balance and strength, stretching, body awareness, decision-making, and targeted core and trunk control seem to reduce modifiable knee injury risk factors by decreasing landing forces, decreasing varus/valgus moments, and increasing effective muscle activation.[61] A plyometric exercise program should be implemented beginning with slow, controlled movements such as stepping up on a platform to faster, more explosive action such as jumping and landing.[59]

Phase 4: Sports-Specific Activities

From 9 to 18 months after surgery, the goal of the rehabilitation is to implement sports-specific activity and eventually return to competition. The timing of anticipated return to play will vary depending on patient-, lesion-, comorbid-, and sports-specific factors, but the athlete may not return before 9 months after ACI. The athlete should continue lower extremity strength training, core strengthening, and plyometric exercises. The athlete may begin a running program that may progress in duration and intensity over the course of the rehabilitation. The athlete should also focus on agility exercises that are specific to the sport of interest. When the patient is able to perform sports-specific activities without pain, he or she may be introduced into limited game situations. General guidelines are that low-impact sports such as swimming, skating, rollerblading, and cycling are permitted at about 9 months, higher-impact sports such as jogging and running at 9 to 12 months, and high-impact sports such as baseball, football, basketball, and tennis between 12 and 18 months.[62]

RETURN TO PLAY AFTER ACI

The duration of rehabilitation after ACI can vary depending on the individual patient, location of the ACI, concomitant procedures, and the type of sport. The appropriate recommendation for return to play can be difficult to ascertain from the literature because there are multiple factors that may lead an athlete to return to competition. In the series by Mithofer and colleagues[8] it was reported that whereas 72% reported good to excellent knee function, only 33% were able to return to soccer; however, 10 of 12 (83%) high-skill soccer players compared with only 5 of 31 (16%) recreational soccer players were able to return to the same level of competition. The mean time to return to soccer for high-skill players was 14.2 months. The disproportionate percentage of high-level athletes returning to the same level of competition has also been observed in patients undergoing microfracture surgery, with greater than 75% returning to play.[11,63] Some studies have reported that patients who underwent ACI or second-generation ACI have been active in competition for a longer period of time compared with athletes who underwent microfracture, suggesting that autologous chondrocyte implantation may provide a more durable treatment option.[8,11,63,64] There are several factors associated with high-level athletes returning to sports, including a younger age, shorter duration of symptoms, and improved postoperative rehabilitation.[8,11] In addition, there are psychosocial factors that may contribute to whether the patient ultimately returns to the same level of competition, as professional athletes have a socioeconomic incentive to return to play.

SUMMARY

The treatment of cartilage defects in the knee with ACI has been demonstrated to be a good treatment option for an athletic patient population. Although there are only a few studies that have looked at such a population, there are several factors that have been associated with a higher likelihood of return to play: younger age, less than 1 year of symptom duration, isolated lesion, and higher level of competition. Rehabilitation after ACI surgery is based on the biologic incorporation of the graft, graft location, and other concomitant procedures that are performed in the athlete. At 3 months, the athlete should have full range of motion with closed chain muscle strengthening. Between 6 and 9 months, the athlete should have full, pain-free range of motion, and a continuation of strength and conditioning with implementation of a core strengthening and a plyometrics program. The anticipated return to sports may vary depending on comorbidities and the patient-, lesion-, and sports-specific factors, but the athlete may not return earlier than 9 months and may take 12 to 18 months before a return to the same level of competition is possible. Careful, supervised rehabilitation with appropriate expectations should allow the athlete a safe and effective return to play that may provide a longer athletic career and a knee that is durable beyond the playing field.

REFERENCES

1. Jones D, Peterson L. Autologous chondrocyte implantation. J Bone Joint Surg Am 2006;88:2502–20.
2. Curl WW, Krome J, Gordon ES, et al. Cartilage injuries: a review of 31,516 knee arthroscopies. Arthroscopy 1997;13(4):456–60.
3. Walczak BE, McCulloch PC, Kang RW, et al. Abnormal findings on knee magnetic resonance imaging in asymptomatic NBA players. J Knee Surg 2008;21:27–33.
4. Major NM, Helms CA. MR imaging of the knee: findings in asymptomatic collegiate basketball players. AJR Am J Roentgenol 2002;179:641–4.
5. Kaplan LD, Schurhoff MR, Selesnick H, et al. Magnetic resonance imaging of the knee in asymptomatic professional basketball players. Arthroscopy 2005;21: 557–61.
6. LaPrade RF, Burnett QM 2nd, Veenstra MA, et al. The prevalence of abnormal magnetic resonance imaging findings in asymptomatic knees. With correlation of magnetic resonance imaging to arthroscopic findings in symptomatic knees. Am J Sports Med 1994;22:739–45.
7. Eckstein F, Lemberger B, Gratzke C, et al. In vivo cartilage deformation after different types of activity and its dependence on physical training status. Ann Rheum Dis 2005;64:291–5.
8. Mithofer K, Peterson L, Mandelbaum BR, et al. Articular cartilage repair in soccer players with autologous chondrocyte transplantation: functional outcome and return to competition. Am J Sports Med 2005;33:1639–46.
9. Micheli L, Curtis C, Shervin N. Articular cartilage repair in the adolescent athlete: is autologous chondrocyte implantation the answer? Clin J Sport Med 2006;16: 465–70.
10. Kocher MS, Micheli LJ, Yaniv M, et al. Functional and radiographic outcome of juvenile osteochondritis dissecans of the knee treated with transarticular arthroscopic drilling. Am J Sports Med 2001;29:562–6.
11. Blevins FT, Steadman JR, Rodrigo JJ, et al. Treatment of articular cartilage defects in athletes: an analysis of functional outcome and lesion appearance. Orthopedics 1998;21:761–7 [discussion: 767–8].
12. Kish G, Modis L, Hangody L. Osteochondral mosaicplasty for the treatment of focal chondral and osteochondral lesions of the knee and talus in the athlete. Rationale, indications, techniques, and results. Clin Sports Med 1999;18:45–66, vi.
13. Takahara M, Ogino T, Sasaki I, et al. Long term outcome of osteochondritis dissecans of the humeral capitellum. Clin Orthop Relat Res 1999;(363):108–15.
14. Mithofer K, Minas T, Peterson L, et al. Functional outcome of knee articular cartilage repair in adolescent athletes. Am J Sports Med 2005;33:1147–53.

15. Bjordal JM, Arnly F, Hannestad B, et al. Epidemiology of anterior cruciate ligament injuries in soccer. Am J Sports Med 1997;25:341–5.
16. Peterson L, Minas T, Brittberg M, et al. Two- to 9-year outcome after autologous chondrocyte transplantation of the knee. Clin Orthop Relat Res 2000;(374):212–34.
17. Jones G, Bennell K, Cicuttini FM. Effect of physical activity on cartilage development in healthy kids. Br J Sports Med 2003;37:382–3.
18. Hefti F, Beguiristain J, Krauspe R, et al. Osteochondritis dissecans: a multicenter study of the European Pediatric Orthopedic Society. J Pediatr Orthop B 1999;8:231–45.
19. Peterson L, Minas T, Brittberg M, et al. Treatment of osteochondritis dissecans of the knee with autologous chondrocyte transplantation: results at two to ten years. J Bone Joint Surg Am 2003;85(Suppl 2):17–24.
20. Minas T. The role of cartilage repair techniques, including chondrocyte transplantation, in focal chondral knee damage. Instr Course Lect 1999;48:629–43.
21. Mandelbaum B, Browne J, Fu F, et al. Articular cartilage lesions of the knee. Current concepts. Am J Sports Med 1998;26:853–61.
22. Pascual-Garrido C, Slabaugh MA, L'Heureux DR, et al. Recommendations and treatment outcomes for patellofemoral articular cartilage defects with autologous chondrocyte implantation. Prospective evaluation at average 4-year follow-up. Am J Sports Med 2009;37(Suppl 1):33S–41S.
23. McNickle AG, L'Heureux DR, Yanke AB, et al. Outcomes of autologous chondrocyte implantation in a diverse patient population. Am J Sports Med 2009;37(7):1344–50.
24. Zaslav K, Cole BJ, Brewster R, et al. A prospective study of autologous chondrocyte implantation in patients with failed prior treatment for articular cartilage defects of the knee. Am J Sports Med 2008;36:1–14.
25. Peterson L, Brittberg M, Kiviranta I, et al. Autologous chondrocyte transplantation. Biomechanics and long-term durability. Am J Sports Med 2002;30(1):2–12.
26. Manning WK, Bonner WM Jr. Isolation and culture of chondrocytes from human adult articular cartilage. Arthritis Rheum 1967;10(3):235–9.
27. Grande DA, Pitman MI, Peterson L, et al. The repair of experimentally produced defects in rabbit articular cartilage by autologous chondrocyte transplantation. J Orthop Res 1989;7(2):208–18.
28. Smith AV. Survival of frozen chondrocytes isolated from cartilage of adult mammals. Nature 1965;205:782–4.
29. Ateshian GA, Soslowsky LJ, Mow VC. Quantitation of articular surface topography and cartilage thickness in knee joints using stereophotogrammetry. J Biomech 1991;24(8):761–76.
30. Grande DA, Singh IJ, Pugh J. Healing of experimentally produced lesions in articular cartilage following chondrocyte transplantation. Anat Rec 1987;218(2):142–8.
31. Breinan HA, Minas T, Hsu HP, et al. Effect of cultured autologous chondrocytes on repair of chondral defects in a canine model. J Bone Joint Surg Am 1997;79(10):1439–51.
32. Brittberg M, Nilsson A, Lindahl A, et al. Rabbit articular cartilage defects treated with autologous cultured chondrocytes. Clin Orthop Relat Res 1996;(326):270–83.
33. Minas T, Chiu R. Autologous chondrocyte implantation. Am J Knee Surg 2000;13:41–50.

34. Gillogly SD, Voight M, Blackburn T. Treatment of articular cartilage defects of the knee with autologous chondrocyte implantation. J Orthop Sports Phys Ther 1998; 28:241–51.
35. Alford AJ, Cole BJ. Cartilage restoration, part 2, techniques, outcomes, and future directions. Am J Sports Med 2005;33(3):443–60.
36. O'Driscoll SW, Keeley FW, Salter RB. The chondrogenic potential of free autogenous periosteal grafts for biological resurfacing of major full-thickness defects in joint surfaces under the influence of continuous passive motion. An experimental investigation in the rabbit. J Bone Joint Surg Am 1986;68(7):1017–35.
37. Reinold MM, Wilk KE, Macrina LC, et al. Current concepts in the rehabilitation following articular cartilage repair procedures in the knee. J Orthop Sports Phys Ther 2006;36(10):774–94.
38. Robertson WB, Gilbey H, Ackland T. Standard practice exercise rehabilitation protocols for matrix induced autologous chondrocyte implantation femoral condyles. Perth (Western Australia): Hollywood Functional Rehabilitation Clinic; 2004.
39. Hambly K, Bobic V, Wondrasch B, et al. Autologous chondrocyte implantation postoperative care and rehabilitation: science and practice. Am J Sports Med 2006;34(6):1020–38.
40. Minas T, Peterson L. Advanced techniques in autologous chondrocyte transplantation. Clin Sports Med 1999;18:13–44, v–vi.
41. Ebert JR, Robertson WB, Lloyd DG, et al. Traditional vs accelerated approaches to post-operative rehabilitation following matrix-induced autologous chondrocyte implantation (MACI): comparison of clinical, biomechanical and radiographic outcomes. Osteoarthritis Cartilage 2008;16(10):1131–40.
42. Wood D, Zheng M, Robertson B. An Australian experience of ACI and MACI. In: Bentley G, editor. Current developments in autologous chondrocyte implantation, round table series, vol. 77. London: Royal Society of Medicine Press Ltd; 2003. p. 7–16.
43. Patel VV, Hall K, Ries M, et al. A three-dimensional MRI analysis of knee kinematics. J Orthop Res 2004;22(2):283–92.
44. McGinty G, Irrgang JJ, Pezzullo D. Biomechanical considerations for rehabilitation of the knee. Clin Biomech (Bristol, Avon) 2000;15(3):160–6.
45. Martelli S, Pinskerova V. The shapes of the tibial and femoral articular surfaces in relation to tibiofemoral movement. J Bone Joint Surg Br 2002;84(4):607–13.
46. Grelsamer RP, Klein JR. The biomechanics of the patellofemoral joint. J Orthop Sports Phys Ther 1998;28(5):286–98.
47. Lee TQ, Morris G, Csintalan RP. The influence of tibial and femoral rotation on patellofemoral contact area and pressure. J Orthop Sports Phys Ther 2003;33(11): 686–93.
48. McConnell J. The physical therapist's approach to patellofemoral disorders. Clin Sports Med 2002;21(3):363–87.
49. Powers CM, Ward SR, Fredericson M, et al. Patellofemoral kinematics during weight-bearing and non-weight-bearing knee extension in persons with lateral subluxation of the patella: a preliminary study. J Orthop Sports Phys Ther 2003; 33(11):677–85.
50. Cohen NP, Foster RJ, Mow VC. Composition and dynamics of articular cartilage: structure, function, and maintaining healthy state. J Orthop Sports Phys Ther 1998;28(4):203–15.
51. Irrgang JJ, Pezzullo D. Rehabilitation following surgical procedures to address articular cartilage lesions in the knee. J Orthop Sports Phys Ther 1998;28(4): 232–40.

52. Fuchs S, Thorwesten L, Niewerth S. Proprioceptive function in knees with and without total knee arthroplasty. Am J Phys Med Rehabil 1999;78:39–45.
53. Ericson MO, Nisell R. Patellofemoral joint forces during ergometric cycling. Phys Ther 1987;67:1365–9.
54. Baker V, Bennell K, Stillman B, et al. Abnormal knee joint position sense in individuals with patellofemoral pain syndrome. J Orthop Res 2002;20:208–14.
55. Fremerey RW, Lobenhoffer P, Zeichen J, et al. Proprioception after rehabilitation and reconstruction in knees with deficiency of the anterior cruciate ligament: a prospective, longitudinal study. J Bone Joint Surg Br 2000;82:801–6.
56. Hess T, Gleitz M, Hopf T, et al. Changes in muscular activity after knee arthrotomy and arthroscopy. Int Orthop 1995;19:94–7.
57. Leetun DT, Ireland ML, Willson JD, et al. Core stability measures as risk factors for lower extremity injury in athletes. Med Sci Sports Exerc 2004;36(6):926–34.
58. Richardson CA, Jull GA. Muscle control-pain control: what exercises would you prescribe? Man Ther 1995;1:2–10.
59. Wilson JD, Dougherty CP, Ireland ML, et al. Core stability and its relationship to lower extremity function and injury. J Am Acad Orthop Surg 2005;13(5):316–25.
60. Hewett TE. ACL injury prevention programs. In: Hewett TE, Shultz SJ, Griffin LY, editors. Understanding and preventing non-contact ACL injuries. 1st edition. Champaign (IL): Human Kinetics; 2007. p. 57–60.
61. Alentorn-Geli E, Myer GD, Silvers HJ, et al. Prevention of non-contact anterior cruciate ligament injuries in soccer players. Part 2: a review of prevention programs aimed to modify risk factors and to reduce injury rates. Knee Surg Sports Traumatol Arthrosc 2009;17:859–79.
62. Gillogly SD, Myers TH, Reinhold MM. Treatment of full-thickness chondral defects in the knee with autologous chondrocyte implantation. J Orthop Sports Phys Ther 2006;36(10):751–64.
63. Steadman JR, Miller BS, Karas SG, et al. The microfracture technique in the treatment of full-thickness chondral lesions of the knee in National League Football players. J Knee Surg 2003;16:83–6.
64. Kon E, Gobbi A, Filardo G, et al. Arthroscopic second-generation autologous chondrocyte implantation compared with microfracture for chondral lesions of the knee: prospective nonrandomized study at 5 years. Am J Sports Med 2009;37(1):33–41.

Rehabilitation of the Knee After Medial Patellofemoral Ligament Reconstruction

Donald C. Fithian, MD[a,b,c,*], Christopher M. Powers, PhD, PT[d,e], Najeeb Khan, MD[b,c]

KEYWORDS

- Medial patellofemoral ligament • Reconstruction
- Rehabilitation • Exercise • Lower limb

Rehabilitation of the extensor mechanism after patellar stabilization surgery should be based on a sound understanding of lower limb mechanics, anatomy, mechanics of the injured or repaired extensor mechanism, and a careful evaluation of the patient. Abnormal anatomic features and control deficits can, and often do, affect function of the patellofemoral joint. Current evidence suggests that patellofemoral rehabilitation should address dynamic lower extremity function, such as abnormal lower extremity motions stemming from impairments proximally (ie, hip) or distally (ie, foot), because such motions can influence the dynamic quadriceps angle (Q-angle) (**Fig. 1**).[1] In addition, many patients with episodic patellar instability have preexisting anatomic deficiencies that may affect rehabilitation.[2] Joint surface injury and degenerative articular lesions also may call for variations to the rehabilitation protocol. The purpose of this article is to provide the reader with an understanding of the current state of lower limb rehabilitation for patients who have undergone medial patellofemoral ligament (MPFL) reconstruction.

Conflict of Interest: Dr Powers acknowledges a financial interest in the SERF Strap that was mentioned in this paper.

[a] Southern California Permanente Medical Group, San Diego, CA, USA
[b] Department of Orthopedic Surgery, Kaiser Permanente, 250 Travelodge Drive, El Cajon, CA 92020, USA
[c] San Diego Knee and Sports Medicine Fellowship, San Diego, CA, USA
[d] Musculoskeletal Biomechanics Research Laboratory, University of Southern California, Los Angeles, CA, USA
[e] Program in Biokinesiology, Division of Biokinesiology & Physical Therapy, University of Southern California, 1540 East Alcazar Street, CHP 155, Los Angeles, CA 90089-9006, USA
* Corresponding author. Department of Orthopedic Surgery, Kaiser Permanente, 250 Travelodge Drive, El Cajon, CA 92020.
E-mail address: donald.c.fithian@kp.org (D.C. Fithian).

Clin Sports Med 29 (2010) 283–290
doi:10.1016/j.csm.2009.12.008 **sportsmed.theclinics.com**

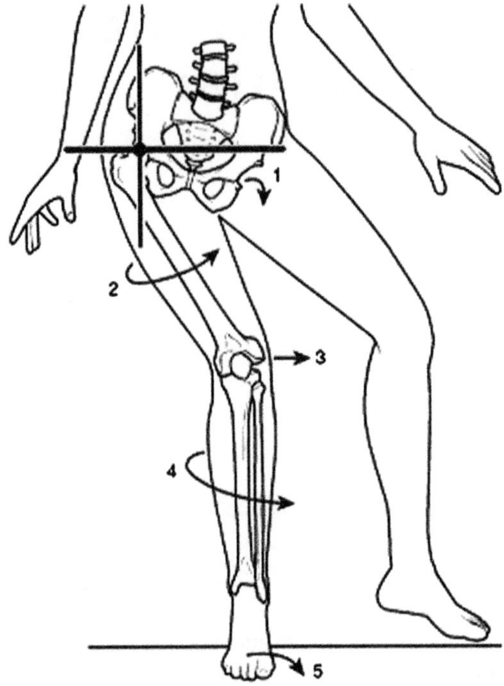

Fig. 1. A diagrammatic representation of the various potential contributions of limb malalignment and malrotation to increase Q-angle: (1) hip adduction, (2) femoral internal rotation, (3) genu valgum, (4) tibial external rotation, and (5) foot pronation. (*From* Powers CM. The influence of altered lower-extremity kinematics on patellofemoral joint dysfunction: a theoretical perspective. J Orthop Sports Phys Ther 2003;33(11):644; with permission.)

PAIN AND SWELLING

MPFL reconstruction is a painful procedure. Severe postoperative pain can interfere with active muscle control. Pain can also impede progress with range of motion (ROM). Operating at or near the medial epicondyle of the knee often is associated with postoperative stiffness because of the higher degrees of motion of the injured soft tissues relative to the femur during knee flexion and extension. It is important to address this tendency aggressively in the early postoperative phase to avoid stiffness. Once the motion has been established, medial pain and knee stiffness caused by scarring at the femoral attachment of the graft are rare problems.

Swelling, either as free intra-articular fluid (effusion) or as soft tissue edema, also can interfere with joint motion. In addition, effusion inhibits quadriceps function[3] and may be harmful to intra-articular structures, such as articular cartilage.

Both pain and swelling can be addressed in various ways. Strict elevation of the limb and limited activity in the first 1 to 2 days postoperation allow the acute inflammatory phase to pass without further perturbation by overaggressive therapy. During that time, cold therapy may be helpful, whether in the form of ice packs or commercially available cold therapy units. The use of cold therapy to reduce local pain, inflammation, and swelling is a traditional mainstay of treatment after injury.

ROM

Prolonged joint immobilization results in the loss of ground substance and dehydration of the extracellular matrix.[4,5] These changes reduce the distance between fibers within the matrix, causing friction and adhesion that reduce suppleness in periarticular ligaments and cartilage. In contrast, mobilization of an injured joint is associated with enhanced collagen synthesis and more optimal fiber realignment within the tissues, reversing the processes seen with immobilization.

It is not always possible to move joints immediately after surgery, but early motion is clearly desirable.[6] Experience has shown that immediate, controlled ROM is not detrimental to fixation or graft development in well-positioned and securely fixed ACL grafts. Furthermore, early motion seems to be beneficial to the limb as a whole by reducing pain, promoting healthy development of cartilage and periarticular tissues, and preventing scar formation and capsular contractions.[7] Therefore 1 goal of MPFL reconstruction is to use a competent graft, place it so that it will not be harmed by physiologic motion, and secure it well enough to withstand the loads associated with normal joint motion.

After MPFL reconstruction, loss of full passive extension is rarely seen. However, it can be difficult to regain full flexion. In addition, failure to achieve full active extension (residual extensor lag) has been reported at short and long-term follow-up.[8] The reasons for motion difficulties after MPFL reconstruction seem to be related to the dissection and MPFL graft location. Cyclops lesions, such as those that can physically block knee extension after ACL reconstruction, have not been reported after MPFL reconstruction. But capsular and/or infrapatellar fat pad contracture, quadriceps inhibition, and poorly positioned grafts can lead to the complications noted earlier.

An early goal of rehabilitation after MPFL reconstruction is to reestablish full knee extension. Unlike ACL reconstruction, return of passive knee extension does not guarantee full active extension. For that to occur, attention must focus on quadriceps strengthening (see later discussion for details). Pain and swelling can be mitigated with electrical stimulation, cold therapy, and compression wraps. Passive patellar glides should be instituted as soon as tolerated, to reestablish normal passive patellar mobility within the trochlear groove in all directions (superiorly, inferiorly, medially, and laterally). Many patients have considerable apprehension because of their prior experience with patellar hypermobility, and mobilization can improve confidence in their newly acquired patella stability.

Return of passive flexion can be difficult for several reasons. If the graft is not positioned properly it may tighten in flexion and tether the joint. Injury around the medial epicondyle, whether traumatic or surgical, is also associated with persistent joint stiffness if early attention is not given to full knee flexion in the rehabilitation program. The goal is to exceed 90° flexion within 6 weeks postoperatively. If that goal is achieved, then in the authors' experience limited knee flexion will not be a problem. On the other hand, delay in achieving greater than 90° of knee flexion may allow scar tissue proliferation and formation of adhesions around the graft and within the medial knee soft tissues. Manipulation may be required to regain full knee motion if flexion past 90° is not accomplished by week 6.

QUADRICEPS STRENGTHENING

Surgery of the extensor mechanism is particularly prone to cause quadriceps inhibition and dysfunction, and every effort should be made to regain quadriceps control, strength, and endurance. If the reconstruction has been performed properly, then controlled quadriceps contractions pose no threat to the graft. Quadriceps setting exercises should be started immediately after the surgery to keep the patellar tendon and infrapatellar fat pad stretched to their full length and to restore neuromuscular control. Resisted quadriceps and hamstring strengthening should be progressively used as the initial pain subsides.

A strong body of levels 1 and 2 studies indicates that electrical stimulation is helpful in reducing strength loss after knee ligament surgery. Classic studies on rehabilitation after ACL reconstruction have demonstrated the value of electrical stimulation compared with voluntary contractions alone for reducing postoperative abnormalities of gait and strength.[9–11] These earlier studies are supported by recent works, indicating that electrical stimulation combined with voluntary exercises is superior to voluntary exercises alone in restoring normal gait and strength.[12] A recent review of these studies recommended neuromuscular electrical stimulation in combination with volitional contraction. Previous investigators have emphasized early application of this approach, when muscle inhibition is most pronounced, to gain maximum effect.[7] Despite differences between MPFL and ACL reconstruction surgeries, there are enough similarities in postoperative neuromuscular deficiencies to suggest that strategies that are found to be successful after ACL reconstruction should be considered for those who have undergone MPFL reconstruction.

WEIGHT BEARING

MPFL reconstruction, whether performed alone or in combination with osteotomy of the tibial tubercle, is not affected by axial loading of the joint. For this reason, there should be no a priori reason to limit weight bearing after surgery as long as axial rotation of the limb is not allowed. The limb should be splinted in a brace during weight-bearing activities for 4 to 6 weeks postoperatively or at least until limb control is sufficient to prevent falls and rotational stress on the knee. Early weight bearing should follow a gradual progression from full protection with a rigid brace locked at full extension to an unlocked brace with crutches. Gradual increase to full weight bearing should be permitted as quadriceps strength is restored.

Care should be taken during weight bearing to prevent dynamic knee valgus and hip internal rotation, which can cause abnormal loads on the healing graft. This is important because many patients with patellofemoral disorders have preexisting deficiencies in proximal limb control that can contribute to these motions.[1,13,14] When postoperative quadriceps weakness and neuromuscular inhibition is superimposed on poor proximal control, unprotected weight bearing can result in abnormal forces on the healing graft. A frequently cited study of graft healing in dogs suggested that 8 to 12 weeks are required for tendon-to-bone healing within tunnels to support graft tension without the risk of slippage.[15] For this reason, care is needed to avoid any rotational activity during the first 3 months postoperatively. Unprotected single-leg stance on the operated knee should be avoided until satisfactory proximal limb control has been achieved. The postoperative brace should be removed for resisted flexion and extension strengthening as well as other controlled rehabilitative exercises that do not cause knee valgus or axial rotational torque that would jeopardize the graft fixation.

Treatment to enhance proximal control can be started preoperatively and then immediately after surgery. Postoperatively, patients should perform non–weight bearing exercises targeting the hip abductors, external rotators, and extensors. When performing strengthening exercises for the gluteus medius, the patient must take care to minimize the contribution of the tensor fascia lata, because contraction of this muscle contributes to medial rotation of the lower extremity. Once the patient is able to isolate the proximal muscles of interest in non–weight bearing exercises, progression to weight-bearing activities can begin.

Facilitation of normal gait is an essential component of the overall treatment plan. This is particularly important for the returning athlete (especially runners), in whom even a slight gait deviation can be compounded by repetitive loading. The clinician should pay particular attention to the quadriceps avoidance gait pattern (walking with the knee extended or hyperextended). Because knee flexion during weight acceptance is critical for shock absorption,[16] this key function must be restored to prevent the deleterious effects of high-impact tibiofemoral joint loading.

The primary causes of quadriceps avoidance are pain, effusion, and quadriceps muscle weakness. As these impairments are addressed in other aspects of treatment, the clinician should keep in mind that resolution of symptoms may not readily translate into a normalized gait pattern. This is particularly evident in a patient with long-term pain and dysfunction. Movement patterns can be learned, and the patient may need to be reeducated with respect to key gait deficiencies. Electromyographic (EMG) biofeedback can be an effective tool for this purpose (**Fig. 2**).

DYNAMIC LIMB STABILIZATION AND CONTROL

Functional training of the limb can begin in earnest 3 months after surgery. At this time, the patient should be introduced to the concept of neutral lower extremity alignment. This involves alignment of the lower extremity such that the anterior superior iliac spine and knee remain positioned over the second toe, with the hip positioned neutrally

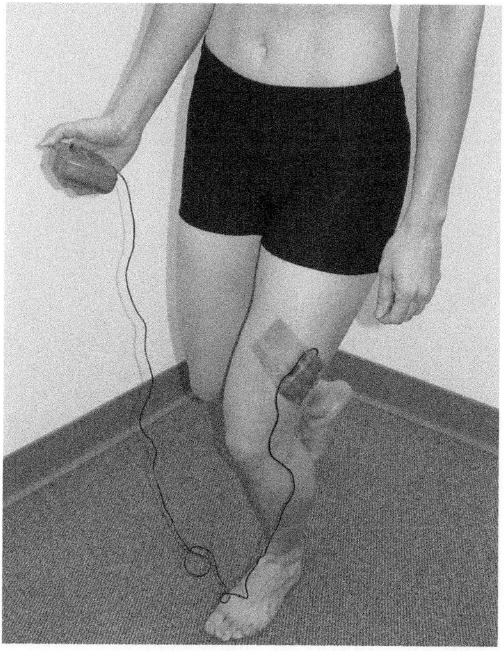

Fig. 2. EMG biofeedback can be used to facilitate quadriceps recruitment during functional tasks. (*Reproduced from* Powers CM, Souza RB, Fulkerson JP. Patellofemoral joint. In: Magee DJ, Zachazewski JE, Quillen WS, editors. Pathology and intervention in musculoskeletal rehabilitation. St. Louis (MO): Saunders Elsevier; 2008. p. 628; with permission.)

(**Fig. 3**). Postural alignment and symmetric strengthening should be emphasized during all exercises (see **Fig. 3**).

If the patient has a difficult time maintaining proper lower extremity alignment during initial weight-bearing exercises, femoral strapping can be used to provide kinesthetic feedback and to augment muscular control and proprioception (**Fig. 4**). Also, taping or bracing of the patellofemoral joint may be done if pain is limiting the patient's ability to engage in a meaningful weight-bearing exercise program. Partial squats, which may have been started already in a controlled environment under supervision, can be advanced to incorporate a BOSU ball (BOSU Fitness LLC, San Diego, CA, USA) or a similar device to facilitate proximal control. Again many patients may exhibit abnormal movements or postures during training tasks. As such close supervision may be necessary to ensure proper execution. Once the patient understands the proper movement and goal of the task, continued performance in front of a mirror provides useful feedback.

As strength, control, and balance progress, single-leg activities may be initiated. This is the final step before returning to full unrestricted activity. Considering that most patients are conditioned by their preoperative apprehension caused by patellar instability and that some patients may not have performed single-leg squats on the operated leg for years before the operation, the patient may not progress to this stage before 5 to 6 months after the reconstruction. In any case, rehabilitation from this point onward requires careful assessment and progressive development of proximal lower limb control.

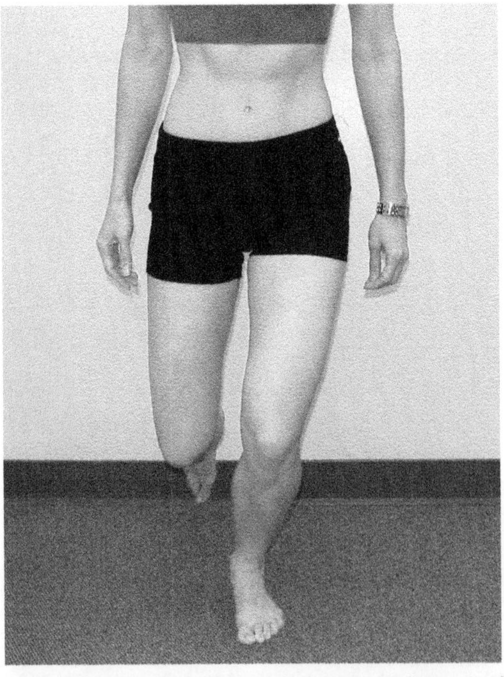

Fig. 3. Weight-bearing activities (such as the single-leg squat shown in the figure) should be done with particular attention to proper alignment of the pelvis, hip, knee, and ankle. (*Reproduced from* Powers CM, Souza RB, Fulkerson JP. Patellofemoral joint. In: Magee DJ, Zachazewski JE, Quillen WS, editors. Pathology and intervention in musculoskeletal rehabilitation. St. Louis (MO): Saunders Elsevier; 2008. p. 631; with permission.)

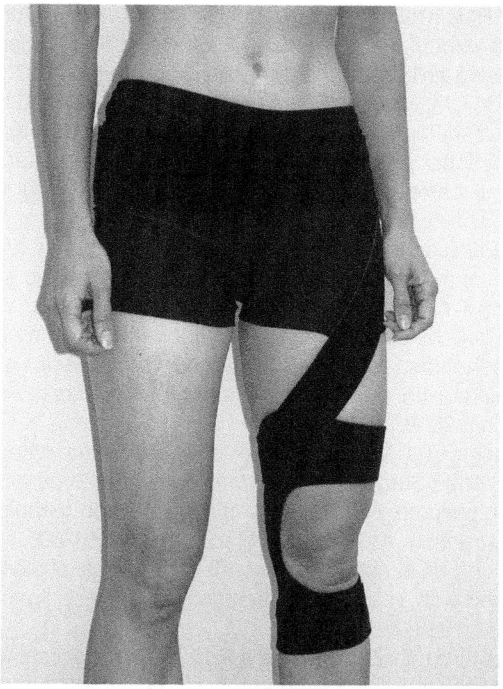

Fig. 4. Femoral strapping (Power Strap, Don Joy Orthopaedics Inc, Carlsbad, CA, USA) can be used to improve lower extremity control and kinematics during the rehabilitation program and functional activities. (*Reproduced from* Powers CM, Souza RB, Fulkerson JP. Patellofemoral joint. In: Magee DJ, Zachazewski JE, Quillen WS, editors. Pathology and intervention in musculoskeletal rehabilitation. St. Louis (MO): Saunders Elsevier; 2008. p. 632; with permission.)

RETURN TO SPORT

Patients should be encouraged to return to their sport or activity gradually once they can achieve satisfactory single limb dynamic control. With competitive or recreational athletes who will be returning to full participation, plyometric training (ie, jump training) should be considered during this phase of the rehabilitation program. As patients, particularly athletes, return to sport activities, repetitive forces applied through the knee joint must be controlled adequately to allow continued healing of the injured or repaired tissues. During an extended time of recovery, such as following knee extensor mechanism surgery, quadriceps and hip muscle strength should be maintained (ie, maintenance program) through careful application of resistive exercises. Experience has shown that patients can expect to return to unrestricted activities by 6 months to 1 year postoperatively.

REFERENCES

1. Powers CM. The influence of altered lower-extremity kinematics on patellofemoral joint dysfunction: a theoretical perspective. J Orthop Sports Phys Ther 2003;33: 639–46.
2. Fithian D, Neyret P, Servien E. Patellar instability: the lyon experience. Tech Knee Surg 2007;6:112–23.

3. Palmieri-Smith RM, Kreinbrink J, Ashton-Miller JA, et al. Quadriceps inhibition induced by an experimental knee joint effusion affects knee joint mechanics during a single-legged drop landing. Am J Sports Med 2007;35:1269–75.
4. Vailas AC, Tipton CM, Matthes RD, et al. Physical activity and its influence on the repair process of medial collateral ligaments. Connect Tissue Res 1981;9:25–31.
5. Noyes FR. Functional properties of knee ligaments and alterations induced by immobilization: a correlative biomechanical and histological study in primates. Clin Orthop Relat Res 1977;123:210–42.
6. Haggmark T, Eriksson E. Cylinder or mobile cast brace after knee ligament surgery. A clinical analysis and morphologic and enzymatic studies of changes in the quadriceps muscle. Am J Sports Med 1979;7:48–56.
7. Manske R, DeCarlo M, Davies G, et al. Anterior cruciate ligament reconstruction: rehabilitation concepts. In: Kibler W, editor. Orthopaedic knowledge update: sports medicine 4. 4th edition. Rosemont (IL): American Academy of Orthopaedic Surgeons; 2009. p. 247–56.
8. Thaunat M, Erasmus PJ. Management of overtight medial patellofemoral ligament reconstruction. Knee Surg Sports Traumatol Arthrosc 2009;17:480–3.
9. Anderson AF, Lipscomb AB. Analysis of rehabilitation techniques after anterior cruciate reconstruction. Am J Sports Med 1989;17:154–60.
10. Wigerstad-Lossing I, Grimby G, Jonsson T, et al. Effects of electrical muscle stimulation combined with voluntary contractions after knee ligament surgery. Med Sci Sports Exerc 1988;20:93–8.
11. Snyder-Mackler L, Ladin Z, Schepsis AA, et al. Electrical stimulation of the thigh muscles after reconstruction of the anterior cruciate ligament. Effects of electrically elicited contraction of the quadriceps femoris and hamstring muscles on gait and on strength of the thigh muscles. J Bone Joint Surg Am 1991;73:1025–36.
12. Beynnon BD, Johnson RJ, Abate JA, et al. Treatment of anterior cruciate ligament injuries, part 2. Am J Sports Med 2005;33:1751–67.
13. Souza RB, Powers CM. Predictors of hip internal rotation during running: an evaluation of hip strength and femoral structure in women with and without patellofemoral pain. Am J Sports Med 2009;37:579–87.
14. Souza RB, Powers CM. Differences in hip kinematics, muscle strength, and muscle activation between subjects with and without patellofemoral pain. J Orthop Sports Phys Ther 2009;39:12–9.
15. Rodeo SA, Arnoczky SP, Torzilli PA, et al. Tendon-healing in a bone tunnel. A biomechanical and histological study in the dog. J Bone Joint Surg Am 1993;75:1795–803.
16. Perry J, Antonelli D, Ford W. Analysis of knee-joint forces during flexed-knee stance. J Bone Joint Surg Am 1975;57:961–7.

Rehabilitation Following High Tibial Osteotomy

Kristopher J. Aalderink, MD, Michael Shaffer, PT, ATC, OCS, Annunziato Amendola, MD*

KEYWORDS

• High tibial osteotomy • Rehabilitation • Physical therapy

Tibial osteotomy is an effective surgical intervention for treating knee malalignment associated with pain or arthrosis in young and active patients. Although the techniques have evolved, the basic principle has been used for many years. The advent of improved fixation devices has allowed for earlier and more aggressive return to activity, resulting in the need for new rehabilitation guidelines that are individualized to patient pathology, expectations, and abilities.

CLINICAL INDICATIONS

Clinical indications for high tibial osteotomy most commonly include a varus standing alignment associated with any of the following:

1. Medial compartment arthrosis in a stable knee (classical indication)
2. Medial compartment arthrosis with associated ligament deficiency and instability (eg, anterior cruciate ligament, posterior cruciate ligament, posterolateral corner, or combined ligament deficiencies)
3. Painful medial knee compartment with associated medial meniscus deficiency, articular cartilage defects requiring resurfacing, or osteochondritis dissecans lesions.

These conditions often require a high tibial osteotomy to unload the affected compartment in either a combined or staged procedure. Indications for tibial osteotomy have expanded over the past several years[1,2] to include minor valgus deformities and sagittal plane instabilities.

PREOPERATIVE PATIENT EDUCATION AND SURGICAL PLANNING

The two most common reasons why high tibial osteotomy may fail are inadequate preparation by the surgeon or inadequate preparation of the patient. Surgeons and

University of Iowa Sports Medicine Center, Department of Orthopaedic Surgery and Rehabilitation, University of Iowa Hospitals and Clinics, 200 Hawkins Drive, Iowa City, IA 52245, USA
* Corresponding author.
E-mail address: ned-amendola@uiowa.edu (A. Amendola).

Clin Sports Med 29 (2010) 291–301
doi:10.1016/j.csm.2009.12.005 sportsmed.theclinics.com
0278-5919/10/$ – see front matter

patients are often reluctant to pursue osteotomy, not only because of the nature of the surgery but also because the rehabilitation process is relatively prolonged compared with procedures such as unicompartmental or even total knee arthroplasty.

Therefore, thorough preoperative surgical planning is equally as important as patient education and should include a detailed discussion of the surgical procedure in addition to the postoperative rehabilitation period. Time should be spent addressing patient goals and expectations before and after surgery. Patient selection is a key factor in achieving a successful outcome. Review of a patient's history should include age, occupation, activity level, and other associated medical conditions. All previous surgical procedures involving the affected knee/extremity are important to document. A history of catching, locking, or other mechanical symptoms may indicate a need for an arthroscopic evaluation before performing the osteotomy.

Physical examination should include an evaluation of the lower limb alignment, gait, patellar tracking, range of motion, ligamentous stability, points of tenderness, and the response to unloading the affected compartment from an applied varus or valgus stress. Particular attention should be paid to any deficits of extension, because these will likely remain postoperatively. Generally, loss of extension is related to the degree of arthrosis of the knee. A flexion contracture of 10° to 15° is a contraindication to osteotomy, unless correctable.

Possible correctable causes of lack of extension can be caused by a "bumper" osteophyte (anterior tibial osteophyte that impinges on intercondylar notch with knee extension), soft tissue contracture, concomitant meniscal pathology (ie, anteriorly flipped bucket handle tear), or extensor mechanism insufficiency. If radiographic evidence shows a bumper osteophyte blocking full extension, the osteophyte should be excised before or at surgery.

Accurate preoperative assessment and technical precision are essential to achieve successful outcomes. Knee radiographs are a key component in the preoperative assessment process. The standard assessment at the authors' institution includes bilateral anteroposterior weight-bearing radiographs taken at full extension, bilateral posteroanterior weight-bearing radiographs at 45° of flexion, lateral and skyline films of the affected leg, and full-length (hip to ankle) standing alignment films. Several measurements are taken from these films to help with preoperative planning (**Fig. 1**). The general principle is to determine the desired postoperative location of the weight-bearing line and thereby calculate the angular correction necessary to achieve this. Care is taken to consider both the coronal and sagittal planes for necessary corrections.

Surgeons should also address potential complications from surgery, including infection, malunion, nonunion, neurovascular injury,[3,4] intra-articular fracture, arthrofibrosis, and complications from anesthesia. The authors advise patients who smoke that bone and wound healing can be significantly delayed by exposure to nicotine,[5,6] and recommend complete cessation before surgery. Many patients are referred for general medical evaluation, optimization, and clearance before surgery. Because surgery is associated with a risk for complications, it is prudent to exhaust nonoperative options, such as the use of heel wedges or unloader braces, Synvisc injections, and activity modification, before operating.

The postoperative period must be clearly outlined for patients, from hospitalization; pain expectations; weight-bearing status; ability to sit, stand, and walk; and, depending on their work, when they can walk, drive, and return to more aggressive activities. Estimates on when to return to work are individualized based on the demands and accommodations that can be made in the work environment. Those who have a desk job may expect to return as soon as 2 to 3 weeks after surgery. More

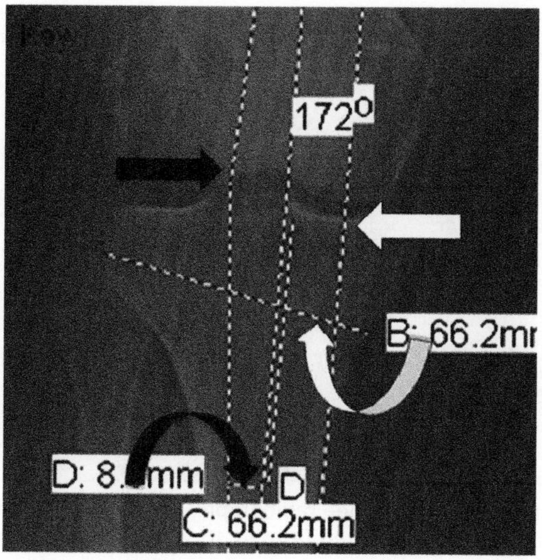

Fig. 1. Anteroposterior knee radiograph showing preoperative alignment calculations and proposed tibial osteotomy. White block arrow, mechanical axis drawn from center of femoral head to center of talus. Black block arrow, desired mechanical axis correction to lateral tibial spine. Curved white arrow, size of wedge needed for desired mechanical axis correction (~8 mm). Curved black arrow, proposed tibial osteotomy trajectory.

labor-intensive occupations may necessitate a longer period before return to work, typically 3 to 4 months. The authors routinely instruct their patients that complete recovery after a high tibial osteotomy, defined as a pain-free return to full activity, including unlimited exercise, can take 6 months or longer. Patients are universally instructed that they will be limited to strictly non–weight-bearing activity for the first 6 weeks after surgery to ensure a stable osteotomy (**Fig. 2**), and that progression will occur at the 6-week evaluation period, pending radiographs that show progressive bony healing.

The postoperative rehabilitative course is integral to the overall success of the operation. Patients must understand the reason for surgery, but more importantly, the rationale for the rehabilitation process. For this reason, the authors' patients meet with a rehabilitation specialist or physical therapist as part of their preoperative consultation. This meeting enables the therapist to review the correct use and function of the postoperative brace and crutches, discuss postoperative precautions, and show appropriate postoperative exercises to be performed between hospital discharge and the first postoperative appointment.

OPERATIVE PROCEDURE

Options for high tibial osteotomy include the traditional opening wedge (typically medial to correct varus malalignment), and closing wedge osteotomy, as popularized by Coventry[7] and Insall and colleagues.[8] Fixation devices have evolved from cylindrical casting, staples, screws, various plate constructs, and many external fixation methods. Acute correction of deformity and plating is preferred for most cases. With large or complex deformities, gradual correction with an external fixator will allow for accurate monitoring of the alignment correction.

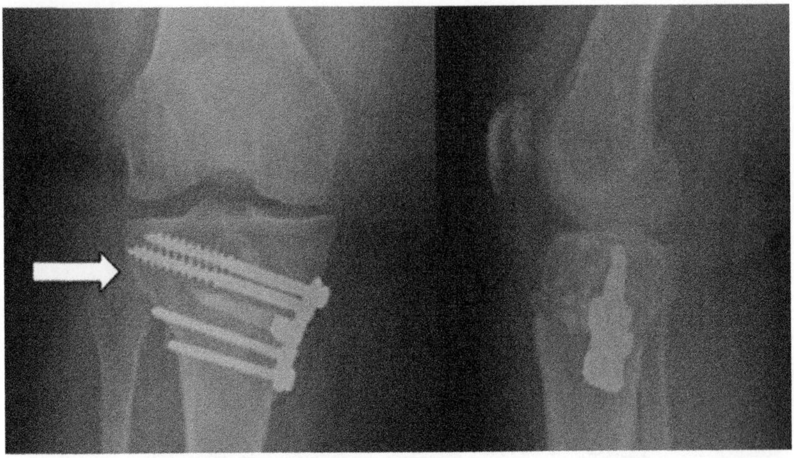

Fig. 2. Anteroposterior and lateral knee radiographs illustrating a stable tibial osteotomy. The lateral cortex has not been violated (*arrow*), thus maintaining alignment in both the coronal and sagittal planes.

Although the lateral closing wedge osteotomy is the most commonly reported osteotomy for treating medial compartment arthrosis, the medial opening wedge osteotomy offers several advantages over a lateral closing wedge osteotomy, as shown in **Box 1**. Theoretically, a medial opening wedge osteotomy restores anatomy with the addition of bone to the diseased medial side, allows for predictable correction in both coronal and sagittal planes with the added ability to adjust the correction intraoperatively, requires only one bone cut, avoids disruption of the proximal tibiofibular joint, and can be easily combined with other procedures. Disadvantages of the opening wedge include the biologic healing capacity of the osteotomy site; stability

Box 1
Advantages and disadvantages of medial opening wedge osteotomy

Advantages

- Restores anatomy
- Allows predictable correction of multiplane deformities (coronal and sagittal planes)
- Requires only one bone cut
- Avoids disruption of tibiofibular joint
- Can be easily combined with other surgical procedures (osteocondritis dessicans allografting, meniscal transplant)

Disadvantages

- Biologic healing capacity of osteotomy site
- More unstable than closing wedge
- Requires protection from weight-bearing initially
- Results in a relative lengthening of the limb

of the construct, which requires protection until some healing has occurred; and the relative lengthening of the limb, which may be noticeable to some patients.

Medial Opening Wedge Osteotomy

Knowledge of the anatomy involved in the surgery is important for physical therapists to understand the recovery from surgery. A 5-cm longitudinal incision is created, extending from 1 cm below the medial joint line midway between the medial border of the tubercle and the posteromedial border of the tibia. The sartorial fascia is exposed through sharp dissection. The superior border of the sartorius fascia is incised and the pes anserinus tendons are retracted distally with a blunt retractor, exposing the superficial fibers of the medial collateral ligament. The anterior border of the medial ligament is identified and raised with a scalpel and periosteal elevator to the posteromedial border of the tibia. A blunt curved retractor is then passed around the posteromedial tibia to protect the posterior neurovascular structures.

Fixation failure and intra-articular fracture is more likely with increased obliquity of the osteotomy and proximity to the lateral tibial plateau. Using guide pins, the tibial osteotomy is performed immediately distal to the guide pin, with the pin protecting against proximal migration of the osteotomy and risk for intra-articular fracture. The osteotomy should be performed above the patellar tendon insertion, with a medial starting position distal enough to allow sufficient bone for positioning of the fixation plate on the proximal fragment. The osteotomy should be at least 1 cm distal to the tibial articular surface at its most proximal (lateral) extent, and directed toward the upper end of the proximal tibiofibular articulation. The slope of the osteotomy in the sagittal plane is critical and should mimic the proximal tibial joint slope.

Alignment should be checked with fluoroscopy intermittently while opening the osteotomy. Once the calculated preoperative correction has been reached, a long alignment rod can be used with fluoroscopy. Attention should be paid to the coronal and sagittal correction to avoid inadvertent changes to the tibial slope. With opening wedge osteotomy the slope tends to increase, whereas with closing wedge osteotomy the slope is generally decreased.

Once the desired correction has been achieved and the plate position determined, the plate is secured with two partially threaded 6.5-mm cancellous screws proximally and two 4.5-mm fully threaded screws distally. Fluoroscopic guidance should be used for the proximal screws to avoid penetration into either the joint or the osteotomy.

The defect is then grafted using cancellous chips in defects less than 7.5 mm. In defects 10 mm or greater, the authors use cancellous chips in the lateral aspect of the defect and two corticocancellous wedges medially, one anterior and one posterior to the plate. Final fluoroscopic assessment ensures adequate position of the osteotomy and hardware and complete filling of the defect with bone graft. In addition, any concerns about the stability of the construct must be assessed because this may affect the progression of rehabilitation.

Lateral Closing Wedge Osteotomy

The goal of a lateral closing wedge osteotomy is correction of alignment, as outlined previously, achieved by removing a laterally based wedge of bone and closing the resultant defect. The skin incision the authors use is L-shaped, with the vertical limb along the lateral edge of the tibial tubercle and the horizontal limb parallel and 1 cm distal to the lateral joint line, taken posteriorly to the anterior aspect of fibular head. Dissection is performed to expose the fascia of the anterior compartment, which is incised along the anterolateral crest of the tibia, leaving a 5-mm cuff for later closure. A Cobb elevator is used to elevate the muscle from the anterolateral surface of the tibia, and the iliotibial tract is elevated from Gerdy's tubercle proximally, inserting a stay suture for retraction and later closure. The common peroneal nerve is not routinely exposed but is palpated and protected throughout the procedure.

Treatment of the proximal tibiofibular joint also has many described techniques, including joint excision or disruption, fibular osteotomy, or excision of the fibular head. The authors prefer to disrupt the joint but preserve the fibular head. The proximal tibiofibular joint is exposed, the anterior capsule incised, and a curved osteotome directed posteromedially to disrupt this articulation and mobilize the fibula so as not to impede later correction. A Z-shaped retractor is placed through this joint along the posterior aspect of the tibia to protect posterior soft tissues. The lateral edge of the patellar tendon is identified, and a second Z retractor placed underneath to protect it during the osteotomy. In this way, the proximal tibia is exposed from tibial tubercle to the posterolateral cortex and is therefore prepared for the osteotomy.

In removing a laterally based wedge, either an angular cutting guide can be used or a specific sized wedge can be removed. The preferred technique is to remove the outer cortex and large portion of the wedge with saw cuts, then remove the medial half using a combination of curettes, rongeurs, and osteotomes before closing the osteotomy. In performing these cuts, the position of anterior and posterior retractors should be checked to ensure soft tissue protection and to cut the anterior and posterior cortices fully, to within 1 cm of the medial cortex. Fluoroscopy can be used to help assess completeness of wedge removal. Once closed, position and alignment are checked with fluoroscopy and fixation is completed; this is usually done with two stepped staples, or alternatively an ASIF L- or T-shaped plate.

POSTOPERATIVE REHABILITATION PROTOCOL

Postoperative rehabilitation is divided into four phases: (I) the immediate in-hospital and home convalescence stage (0–2 weeks), (II) the subacute stage characterized by non–weight-bearing while the osteotomy site heals (2–6 weeks), (III) progressive weight-bearing and strengthening after bone healing (6–12 weeks), and finally (IV) a return to full activities (3–9 months).

Phase I: Initial Postoperative Period (0–2 weeks)

Immediately after surgery, patients are placed in a hinged knee brace locked in full extension. The brace is to be worn at all times, including while sleeping, but is unlocked for in-hospital use of a continuous passive motion machine (CPM). The CPM is used to maintain knee motion and help reduce postoperative swelling. The CPM machine may be continued at home, for 4 to 6 hours per day, if restoring range of motion (ROM) is problematic. However, most patients are able to regain ROM without the home use of a CPM by regularly performing active assisted flexion exercises, such as seated flexion and heel slides (**Fig. 3**).

Patients are encouraged to achieve 90° of knee flexion and full knee extension by the end of the second postoperative week. If extension ROM is problematic, patients may perform prone hangs and prolonged knee extension stretching (extension bridging) for up to 5 minutes at a time (**Fig. 4**). During surgery, increasing the posterior tibial slope (sagittal alignment) must be avoided by placing the plate as far posteromedially as possible. Failure to position the plate posteriorly will leave a larger gap anteriorly, thereby increasing the tibial slope. Patients who lack full extension in the operating room will not achieve full extension postoperatively, regardless of aggressive rehabilitation and stretching.

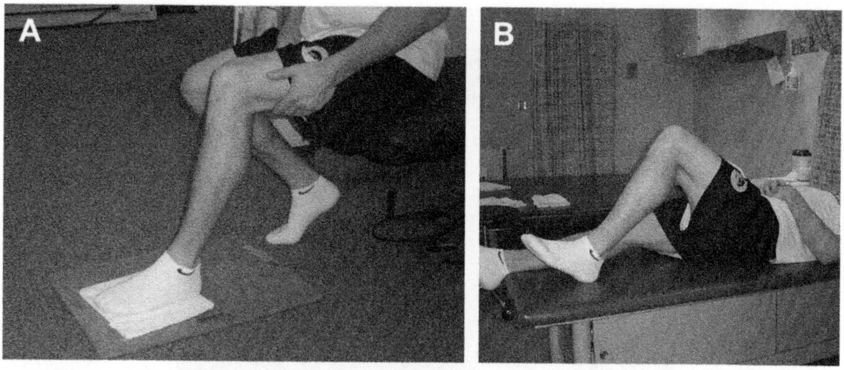

Fig. 3. Active-assisted knee flexion range of motion. (*A*) Seated flexion rarely causes the posterior knee pain often experienced by patients postsurgically when they perform the more common heel slides (*B*).

During the initial two postoperative weeks, the strengthening program consists only of isometric quadriceps femoris contraction (quadriceps sets) performed in full extension.

Patients are instructed to follow strict non–weight-bearing precautions on two axillary crutches with their brace locked in full extension. Finally, patients should ice, elevate, and compress their knee to control postoperative edema. A commercial unit (**Fig. 5**) can be used or patients can use a standard ice pack with an Ace wrap or compressive stockings.

Phase II: Non–weight-Bearing Strengthening (2–6 weeks)

Hip girdle strengthening exercises such as four-plane straight leg raises (**Fig. 6**) are added at 2 weeks postoperatively to advance the strengthening program while maintaining non–weight-bearing status. Terminal extension exercises, such as short arc quad sets, are also implemented around 2 weeks postoperatively (**Fig. 7**). Weight-bearing precautions and crutch training are reviewed at this time because patients are kept non–weight bearing for 6 weeks to allow for bony healing around the osteotomy site.

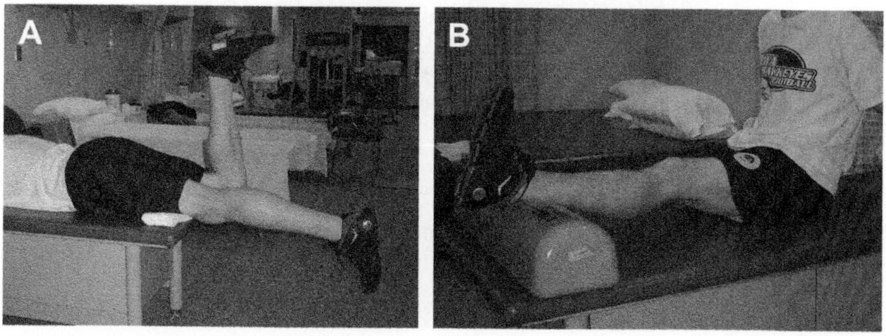

Fig. 4. Exercises such as prone hangs (*A*) and extension bridges (*B*) promote full knee extension through applying a low-load, prolonged stretch.

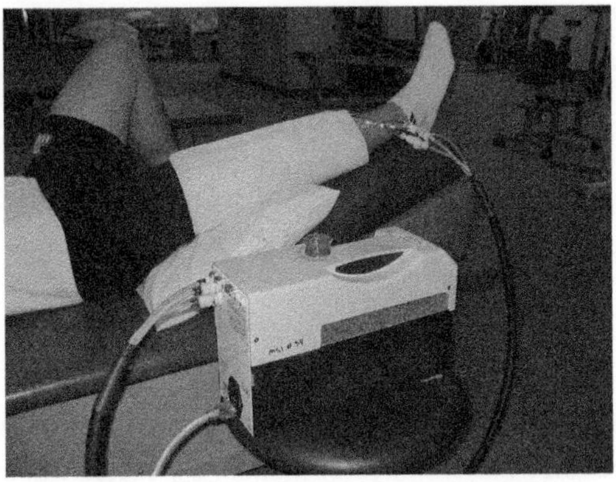

Fig. 5. A commercially available cryotherapy device that allows simultaneous application of cold and compression for managing postoperative edema and pain.

Phase III: Advanced Strengthening and Activity Progression (6–12 weeks)

The progression to weight-bearing is one of the most crucial and often problematic steps in the rehabilitation process. Patients typically fall into one of two categories: those who want to go too fast and bear weight immediately, and those who are cautious and reluctant to bear weight. The physical therapist is an important ally during this transition period, monitoring weight-bearing and assisting with gait training. Protected weight-bearing is critical because the risk for displacement remains as the osteotomy heals. Overzealous activity can result in implant failure and loss of alignment. For unstable osteotomies (**Fig. 8**), patients are kept on crutches for 4 additional weeks after the 6-week visit, and strengthening exercises are delayed until the 10-week mark.

In general, patients are instructed to progress slowly, using pain and swelling as a guide. They are counseled to avoid long periods of standing/walking. The intensity of therapy sessions and rate of progression are reduced if patients experience an increase in osteotomy site pain. Icing for 20 minutes after strenuous activity and each rehabilitation session is an important adjuvant to healing. The goal is to have

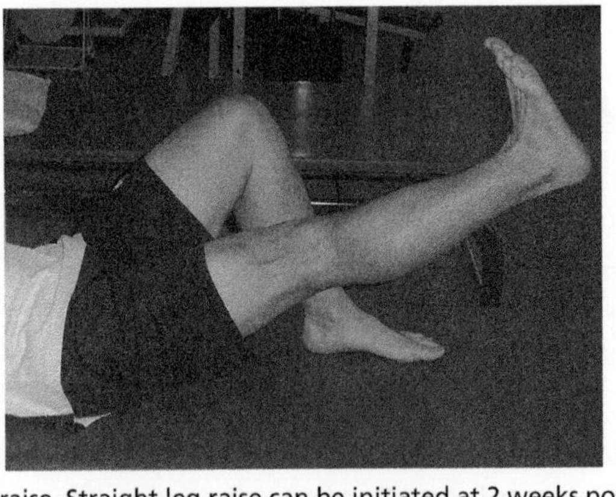

Fig. 6. Straight leg raise. Straight leg raise can be initiated at 2 weeks postoperatively if the patient can easily perform the short-arc quadriceps exercises.

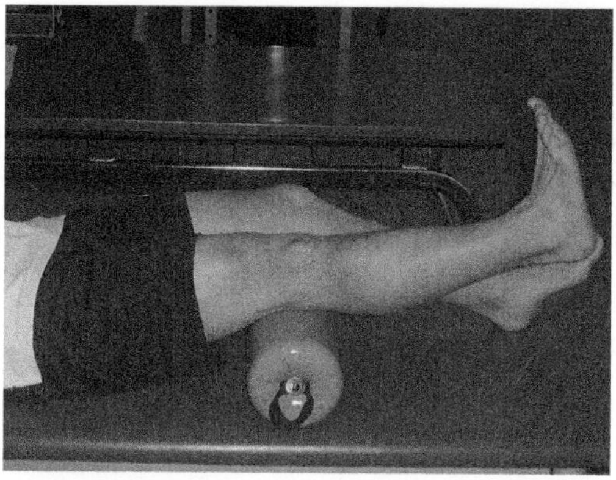

Fig. 7. Short-arc quadriceps exercise. This is a helpful exercise to begin quadriceps strengthening and can be initiated 2 weeks after surgery.

patients ambulating without crutches by 6 to 8 weeks after surgery. Most patients are able to return to normal ambulation (ie, without a limp) at this time.

Phase IV: Return to Activity (3–9 months)

A return to low-impact activities (elliptical, bicycle) typically takes 3 to 4 months, and a return to high-impact activities (running, sports) after 6 months or longer. Patients are advised to progress their activities as their knee allows, monitoring their knee for not only pain around the osteotomy site but also the presence of a knee effusion. Patients are particularly cautioned that they may be stressing their knee excessively if pain lasts longer than 24 hours after an activity. **Table 1** outlines the postoperative rehabilitation protocol used at the authors' institution.

Patients are evaluated in the orthopedic clinic at postoperative weeks 2 and 6, with additional evaluations at 3 and 6 months. A therapist also evaluates rehabilitation progress at these intervals. Depending on individual goals or pathology, patients

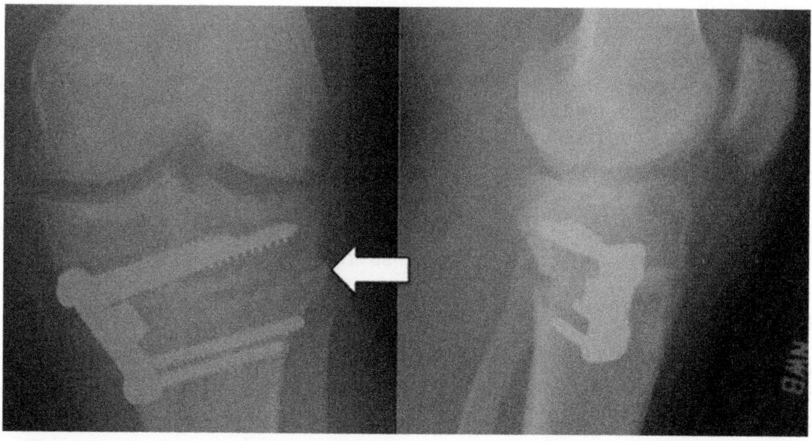

Fig. 8. Anteroposterior and lateral knee radiographs showing an unstable tibial osteotomy. In this example, the lateral tibial cortex has been violated (*arrow*) lending to slight coronal plane (medial-lateral) translation.

Table 1
Postoperative rehabilitation protocol

	Weight-Bearing	Brace	Range of Motion	Therapeutic Exercises
Initial postoperative (0–2 wk)	Non–weight-bearing with crutches	Unlocked from 0°–90°, when seated Locked in full extension when ambulating	0°–90° (2 wk)	ROM: Seated flexion, heel slides, extension bridging Strengthening: Quadriceps sets
Non–weight-bearing strengthening (2–6 wk)	Non–weight-bearing with crutches	Unlocked from 0°–90°, when seated Locked in full extension when ambulating	0°–120° (2–4 wk)	ROM: Hamstring, quad, calf stretching Strengthening: Quadriceps sets, straight leg raise x four directions, non–weight-bearing plantar flexion versus elastic resistance
Advanced strengthening and activity progression (6–12 wk)	Partial weight-bearing, advance to Full weight-bearing	Discontinue brace at 6 wk	Full ROM	ROM: Passive ROM as needed, stationary bicycle Strengthening: Begin mini squats, toe raises, leg press/shuttle, and hamstring curls. CV conditioning: Bicycle, elliptical Proprioception: Single limb stance progression
Return to activity (3–9 mo)	Full weight-bearing			CV conditioning: Bicycle, elliptical, running program (as appropriate): straight ahead jog, run, figure-eights, cutting, sprints, drills Sport-specific training: As appropriate, once all symptoms resolved

may complete their rehabilitation largely independently. However, the key to this approach and to eventually achieving successful rehabilitation postsurgery is to identify and address problems early. If range of motion goals are not met when patients return at the 2-week evaluation, supervised physical therapy sessions are initiated 2 to 3 times per week. In contrast, if patients are having difficulty restoring strength or if problems with the weight-bearing progression are anticipated, supervised therapy may begin at 6 weeks with an emphasis on strengthening and activity progression.

SUMMARY

Tibial osteotomy can successfully alleviate knee pain in the management of malalignment associated with knee arthrosis in young or active patients. Success requires diligence and attention to detail in the operating room. However, a good outcome also depends heavily on thorough preoperative preparation and patient education. Finally, the postoperative rehabilitative course must be closely scrutinized, encouraging steady progress and modifying activities at the completion of each phase of recovery.

REFERENCES

1. Naudie D, Amendola A, Fowler PJ. Opening wedge high tibial osteotomy for symptomatic hyperextension-varus thrust. Am J Sports Med 2004;32(1):60–70.
2. Phisitkul P, Wolf BR, Amendola A. Role of high tibial and distal femoral osteotomies in the treatment of lateral-posterolateral and medial instabilities of the knee. Sports Med Arthrosc 2006;14(2):96–104.
3. Amendola A, Bonasia DE. Results of high tibial osteotomy: review of the literature. Int Orthop 2009. [Epub ahead of print].
4. Georgoulis AD, Makris CA, Papageorgiou CD, et al. Nerve and vessel injuries during high tibial osteotomy combined with distal fibular osteotomy: a clinically relevant anatomic study. Knee Surg Sports Traumatol Arthrosc 1999;7:15–9.
5. Zheng LW, Ma L, Cheung LK. Changes in blood perfusion and bone healing induced by nicotine during distraction osteogenesis. Bone 2008;43(2):355–61.
6. Haverstock BD, Mandracchia VJ. Cigarette smoking and bone healing: implications in foot and ankle surgery. J Foot Ankle Surg 1998;37(1):69–74 [discussion: 78].
7. Coventry MB. Upper tibial osteotomy. Clin Orthop Relat Res 1984;182:46–52.
8. Insall J, Shoji H, Mayer V. High tibial osteotomy: a five-year evaluation. J Bone Joint Surg Am 1974;56:1397–405.

Rehabilitation After Anteromedialization of the Tibial Tuberosity

Nima Salari, MD[a], Gary A. Horsmon, PA-C, ATC[a],
Andrew J. Cosgarea, MD[a,b,*]

KEYWORDS

- Tibial tuberosity • Osteotomy • Rehabilitation
- Anteromedialization • Patellar instability
- Fulkerson osteotomy • Elmslie-Trillat osteotomy

PATHOPHYSIOLOGY AND RATIONALE FOR SURGICAL TREATMENT

Patellar instability is often the result of a traumatic event and occurs more commonly in individuals with imbalances in the static and dynamic stabilizers of the patellofemoral joint. In addition to the risk of recurrent instability, such patients often have suboptimal joint-loading patterns that can lead to damage of the articular surfaces.[1–7] Nonoperative treatment goals guide patients toward performing functional activities without surpassing their optimal joint-loading limits. When nonoperative treatment fails, surgical intervention becomes necessary.

The patellofemoral joint consists of the triangular-shaped patella and its articulation with the femoral condyles. The patella is the longest sesamoid bone in the body and functions as a fulcrum for extension of the leg. Stability of the patellofemoral joint is primarily affected by the bony architecture, particularly by the trochlear ridges, which centralize the patella during knee flexion. Other important static restraints are the medial and lateral patellofemoral ligaments and the retinacula. Besides the lateral trochlear ridge, the medial patellofemoral ligament has been shown to be the key soft-tissue restraint to pathologic lateral displacement of the patella. The quadriceps muscles are the major dynamic stabilizers; of these muscles, the most important is the vastus medialis obliquus (VMO).[6,8,9] Although some patients with recurrent patellar instability are best treated with soft-tissue stabilization procedures (eg, medial patellofemoral ligament repair or reconstruction), this article addresses only bony realignment procedures.

[a] Department of Orthopaedic Surgery, The Johns Hopkins University, Baltimore, MD, USA
[b] Sports Medicine and Shoulder Surgery, The Johns Hopkins Hospital, Baltimore, MD, USA
* Corresponding author. C/o Elaine Henze, Johns Hopkins Bayview Medical Center, 4940 Eastern Avenue, #A665, Baltimore, MD 21224-2780.
E-mail address: ehenze1@jhmi.edu (A.J. Cosgarea).

Clin Sports Med 29 (2010) 303–311
doi:10.1016/j.csm.2009.12.006 sportsmed.theclinics.com

Numerous surgical procedures to treat patients with recurrent patellar instability and symptomatic maltracking have been described. Distal bony realignment operations have been shown to be efficacious with consistently good outcomes and low complication rates.[10–15] The tendency of the patella to dislocate is influenced by numerous factors, including the overall limb alignment and pull of the VMO muscle. The Q-angle, which is measured between a line from the anterior superior iliac spine to the midpatella and a line from the midpatella to the tibial tuberosity, predicts the magnitude of the lateral force vector. The greater the Q-angle, the greater the tendency for the patella to displace laterally and become clinically unstable.[6]

The Elmslie-Trillat (ET) procedure[16] is a popular surgical method for stabilizing the tibial tuberosity, which decreases the Q-angle and improves patellar tracking.[17–19] The tibial tuberosity anteromedialization (AMZ) procedure, popularized by Fulkerson,[18] is another procedure that corrects maltracking by decreasing the Q-angle; in addition, it also decreases the patellofemoral joint reactive forces by concurrently anteriorizing the tibial tuberosity. The AMZ approach, which has become increasingly popular in recent years, is particularly effective for patients with lateral and distal chondral lesions.[2]

SURGICAL INDICATIONS AND TECHNIQUES

To perform distal bony realignment procedures, a shingle of bone surrounding the tibial tuberosity on the proximal tibia is cut, or osteotomized. In the AMZ technique, a transverse cut is made just proximal to the point of attachment of the patellar tendon. A 6-cm shingle is then created by making a longitudinal cut on the bone along the medial edge of the proximal tibial crest. The cut is made from anteromedial to posterolateral and is angled between 30° and 60° in the horizontal plane. The osteotomy converges toward the tibial crest distally, leaving intact a thin area of bone and periosteum. This area serves as a hinge point and remains intact as the proximal portion of the shingle is transferred.

After cutting the bone, the shingle can be moved either directly in the medial direction, as in the ET procedure, or in a combined anterior and medial direction, as in the AMZ procedure. The greater the slope of the cut, the more the shingle is anteriorized as it is medialized. The shingle is usually translated medially approximately 8 to 15 mm, depending on the amount of Q-angle correction that is desired, and hinges off of the intact distal attachment point on the tibial crest. Fixation is achieved with two or three 3.5-mm bicortical screws. The anteriorization component of the translation is particularly important in patients with severe distal chondral and osteochondral lesions. Maquet[17] has shown that patellofemoral forces and pain decrease when the tibial tuberosity is moved anteriorly.

Although the AMZ technique has definite biomechanical advantages over the ET technique in appropriate patients, it requires cutting a larger cross-sectional area of the proximal tibia, which takes longer to heal safely. Patients who undergo the AMZ procedure have a greater risk of postoperative fracture and therefore require a longer period of postoperative protected weight bearing.[3,20] In a cadaveric biomechanical study, Cosgarea and colleagues[3] showed that the tibia was initially more prone to fracturing during AMZ than during the ET procedure. The geometry of the proximal tibia dictates that a larger cross-sectional area of bone is cut with the AMZ technique. The greater the angle of cut, the greater the cross-sectional area of tibia involved in the osteotomy. Because of the risk of fracture, most investigators have recommended restricted or protected weight bearing for 6 weeks or longer in patients undergoing the AMZ procedure.[20–24]

REHABILITATION

Although much has been written on the AMZ surgical technique,[8,15,18] little can be found in the literature regarding rehabilitation and return to activity. As with other surgical procedures, the importance of a rehabilitation program cannot be overemphasized. However, it is vital that all goals are set within the constraints of safe and appropriate guidelines. The key to an early and safe return to activity is a clear, logical, and appropriately aggressive rehabilitation program. A written protocol format can help to organize the process and ease the communication among physicians, therapists, and the patient. The protocol should address the major issues of wound healing, weight bearing, pain, inflammation, swelling, neural inhibition, static and dynamic stabilizers, range of motion, local and systemic neurologic function, proprioception, functional exercises, cardiovascular fitness, and return to activity parameters. Timelines can be created to help provide realistic expectations in terms of range of motion, agility, and strength. However, the protocol must also provide for flexibility because patients vary in terms of motivation, pain tolerance, financial and transportation resources, and ultimate goals. These guidelines are addressed in this article in the following order: (1) treatment of postoperative pain and swelling, (2) weight bearing, (3) restoration of range of motion and normal kinematics, (4) restoration of functional strength and endurance, (5) restoration of proprioception and kinesthetics, (6) restoration of agility progression and running program, (7) restoration of cardiovascular fitness, and (8) return-to-activity guidelines. A protocol that has been formatted in a concise and chronologic fashion (**Table 1**) is provided and can be given to a patient and therapist for an overview of these principles.

Treatment of Postoperative Pain and Swelling

It is imperative that numerous strategies to reduce pain and inflammation are incorporated in the immediate postoperative period. Although these strategies provide a patient with increased comfort, they also enhance a patient's ability to perform efficiently the important range of motion and muscle toning exercises by decreasing apprehension and pain-induced neuromuscular inhibition. Techniques for accomplishing this goal include preemptive analgesia, injection of long-acting local anesthetic in and around the surgical incision, and intraoperative placement of a cryotherapeutic cooling device. Above-the-knee thromboembolic deterrent stockings are applied in the operating room to both the lower extremities to decrease the risks of deep vein thrombosis, surgical-site swelling, and dependent edema.

It is important to manage perioperative pain aggressively with the use of parenteral narcotics in the recovery room. In the authors' experience, virtually all patients can comfortably and safely undergo the AMZ procedure on an outpatient basis. A prescription for oral narcotics to be used in a progressively decreasing fashion for the first 3 to 7 days should be provided on discharge. Most patients start oral nonsteroidal antiinflammatory medications the day after surgery. The authors have also found that the commercially available cryotherapy devices are extremely valuable in modulating pain and swelling and have decreased the need for narcotic pain medication.

After the formal physical therapy program is established, other modalities, such as transcutaneous electrical nerve stimulation, electrical muscle stimulation, ultrasound, and compression, are instituted. Therapeutic techniques involving gentle muscle contractions, elevation, and range of motion for edema reduction and pain control are also used. Compression stockings or tubing can be discontinued after the first few weeks, when most of the swelling has resolved. Most patients use over-the-counter oral analgesics for the first 1 or 2 months to control surgical-site discomfort

Table 1
Tibial tuberosity anteromedialization postoperative rehabilitation protocol

Time Frame	Protocol
Day 1–7	Non–weight-bearing with brace locked in full extension Brace worn 24 hours a day, 7 days a week Quadriceps sets, ankle pumps, straight leg raises Cryotherapy unit, elevation, compression with thromboembolic deterrent stocking
Week 1	Change dressing, check wound Begin supervised physical therapy thrice a week; continue daily home exercise program Unlock brace when in seated or supine position for range of motion exercises Terminal extension exercises Biofeedback, electrical muscle stimulation to assist muscular contraction
Week 2	Sutures removed Anteroposterior and lateral radiographs to include proximal one-third of tibia Ankle weights added to straight leg raises Advance to one-third weight bearing with brace locked in full extension Begin stationary bike for active range of motion
Week 4	Straight leg raises (100 repetitions daily) Advance to two-thirds weight bearing in brace locked in full extension Begin isotonics Partial weight-bearing closed kinetic chain exercises May begin aqua therapy Submaximal isokinetics
Week 6	Advance to full weight bearing in brace locked in full extension Begin early single-leg balance training Increase bike intensity
Week 8	Discontinue brace Should have symmetric range of motion Light elliptical, stairmaster, and treadmill walking
Week 12	Anteroposterior and lateral radiographs to include proximal one-third of tibia Progress to full-speed isotonics and isokinetics Should have approximately 70% strength Initiate progressive running program
Week 16	Should have approximately 80% strength Progress with running speed and distance running Half to three-fourths speed cutting drills Initiate agilities and blind reaction drills
Week 24	Should have approximately 90% strength Sport-specific running, agilities Noncontact practice, if cleared Advance through functional participation Return to sports when cleared by physician

and to maximize the benefits of physical therapy. The authors encourage patients to use their cryotherapy devices as long as the patients think they are beneficial from the perspective of pain modulation.

Weight Bearing

Weight bearing must be limited during the initial stages of recovery not only because the leg muscles are too weak to allow for safe ambulation but also because the osteotomy compromises the structural integrity of the proximal tibia and predisposes it to fracture. The goal of the protocol is to ensure a protected, gradually progressive advancement of weight bearing that safely allows for proper healing of the osteotomy. For the first 2 weeks after surgery, patients are kept non–weight-bearing on crutches while their knees are in a hinged brace locked in full extension. Patients are allowed to progress to one-third weight bearing with crutches after 2 weeks, to two-thirds partial weight bearing with crutches after 4 weeks, and to full weight bearing after 6 weeks. When they are comfortable bearing full weight, they transition off of the crutches. Once the patients exhibit normal gait patterns, the brace is gradually weaned under clinical supervision. Radiographs are obtained and are correlated with the results of clinical examination to confirm that the osteotomy is healing appropriately.

In addition to protecting the healing tibia, the physiologic purposes of these weight-bearing goals are to retrain the individual's close kinetic chain proprioceptive ability and to restore proper gait mechanics. It is essential that patients do not show a limp because doing so can lead to other compensatory musculoskeletal problems. The slow progression also helps patients regain confidence of weight bearing. Weight bearing facilitates soft tissue and bone healing, corrects lower extremity disuse atrophy, and promotes normalization of joint biomechanical function.

Restoration of Range of Motion and Normal Kinematics

Early range of motion exercise has wide-ranging physiologic benefits: it maintains normal kinematics through active, active-assisted, and passive means; contributes to blood flow, pain modulation, prevention of arthrofibrosis, reduction of swelling, and joint proprioception; and instills confidence in the patient regarding the success of the procedure. The entire lower extremity kinetic chain, including the lumbar spine, hip, knee, and ankle joints, must be addressed in the rehabilitation program. The authors' clinical goal is to obtain full symmetric range of motion with the contralateral knee by postoperative week 8. In preparation for weight-bearing exercises, principles of closed kinetic chain are used to assist in functional development of multiple joint-muscle control. Techniques used include active, active-assisted, and passive range of motion; proprioceptive neuromuscular facilitation; terminal extension exercises; and patella mobilizations. For example, active-assisted range of motion involves the therapist assisting the patient, enabling the patient to actively achieve the desired motion. This approach works particularly well for obtaining knee flexion goals.

The principles of proprioceptive neuromuscular facilitation are implemented to help the patient regain range of motion. As the therapist has the patient contract an agonist muscle group (such as the quadriceps), contraction of the antagonist group (the hamstrings) is inhibited. This technique increases hamstring relaxation, improves hamstring stretch, and facilitates knee extension. Examples of gravity-assisted terminal extension exercises are gravity sags (eg, the supine patient props the heel on a pillow) and prone hangs (eg, the prone-lying patient hangs the leg off of the end of a bed). Manual patellar mobilizations are important within the range of the normal soft-tissue constraints, particularly in patients who show early signs of fibrosis or infrapatellar contracture.

Restoration of Functional Strength and Endurance

Efforts at early restoration of dynamic function focus on neuromuscular re-education of the lower extremity musculature, including the quadriceps and, in particular, the VMO. The first goals are reversing of neural inhibition and redeveloping control of muscular contractions, which depend on the successful reduction of postoperative pain and swelling. The process progresses with increasingly intense exercises of all lower extremity muscle groups. Isometrics, isotonics, and isokinetics are used appropriately in the protocol. The benefits of these exercises include increased blood flow, improved proprioception, reduction of disuse atrophy, and reversal of neural inhibition.

Techniques for accomplishing these goals include quadriceps and hamstring sets, 4-way straight leg raises, electrical muscle stimulation, augmented muscular contraction, multiangle isometrics, wall squats, and submaximal isokinetics. Patients then progress from light to heavy isotonics, eccentric contractions, and eventually to full-range isotonics and isokinetics. It is important to include the hip and ankle joints. The most important muscles are the VMO, adductor muscle group, hip flexor muscle group, and hip external rotators. Functional closed kinetic chain resistive exercises (eg, lunges and leg presses) are initiated when appropriate. It is also important to reduce extensor mechanism overload and minimize patellofemoral compression in vulnerable patients by limiting open-chain resisted knee extension exercises. The program should try to incorporate functional speed contractions with the use of isokinetics. Core stabilization is crucial for providing a strong foundation whenever any extremity is being rehabilitated.

Restoration of Proprioception and Kinesthetics

Restoration of local and systemic proprioception and kinesthetic awareness is extremely important for the patient to regain the maximum level of function. This goal is achieved by retraining the postoperative limb and whole body neuromuscular proprioceptive systems to ensure a safe return to functional activities. These exercises start with simple activities, such as balance drills, and progress to more complicated drills, such as plyometrics, kinesthetic coordination drills, and reaction drills. Examples of these drills include rhythmic stabilization, leg ball volleys, minitrampoline use, slide board, deceleration drills, and leg and eye coordination drills. Crawling exercises, which ensure confidence and comfort with patellofemoral weight-bearing activities, may be of benefit to some patients.

Restoration of Agility Progression and Running Program

For individuals who want to return to running and cutting sports, it is necessary to determine the appropriate time to begin that transition. In the authors' experience, most patients are ready to begin treadmill jogging by 3 months. To make the transition, the osteotomy should be healed and patients should have full knee range of motion and approximately 70% of the contralateral leg strength. Strength can be formally measured using an isokinetic dynamometer (such as a Kin-Com [Chattecx Corporation, Chattanooga, TN, USA] or Cybex [Cybex International Inc, Medway, MA, USA] machine), or it can be measured less accurately via manual resistance and functional testing. Slow progression is the key, ranging from endurance walking and biking to elliptical workouts, treadmill workouts, and (eventually) sports surface running. Short-distance progression to develop baseline reconditioning over a period of 1 month should be accomplished before higher intensity running. Slow-speed change-of-direction drills can be incorporated early.

After patient strength improves to approximately 80%, more complex and demanding drills, such as running backward and figure-8 runs, can be incorporated. Ladder drills, carioca runs, dodgeball drills, repetitive single-leg broad jumps, blind reaction drills, and speed drills incorporate the proprioceptive component to this progression. When 90% strength is achieved, sport-specific and game speed drills can be instituted.

Restoration of Cardiovascular Fitness

Comprehensive musculoskeletal rehabilitation necessarily includes the maintenance of cardiovascular conditioning, ultimately to the level of the demand of the sport involved. Use of upper body ergometers allows early cardiovascular conditioning well before the knee is ready to tolerate similar stresses. Partial weight-bearing cardiovascular fitness exercises (eg, stationary bike) may begin as early as 1 month, but full weight-bearing cardiovascular fitness exercises are delayed until 3 months. By 1 to 2 months, it is generally appropriate to progress to swimming, aqua aerobics, and aqua jogging. Implementing accelerated-heart-rate exercise assists with the mental needs of the athlete during rehabilitation and starts to prepare them to resume endurance activities.

Return-to-Activity Guidelines

The ultimate goal of rehabilitation is to enable the athlete to return safely and confidently to the desired level of participation while incorporating all of the physiologic benchmarks of the protocol. This goal is objectively determined not only by simple strength testing but also by the successful completion of sport-specific drills, practice sessions, and complex functional tests. Techniques of functional testing include timed sprints, timed figure-8 runs, measured double- and single-leg broad jump distances, and vertical jump measurements. Successful completion of functional tests requires that the patients display appropriate levels of strength, power, agility, reaction, and proprioception without apprehension, pain, or swelling. A formal return-to-sports clearance is provided to athletes after these goals are met and in consultation with their therapist, trainers, coaches, and parents, when appropriate. Athletes involved in low-risk sports (eg, swimming and biking) may be released to return in as little as 3 months, whereas those involved in higher risk sports (eg, football and lacrosse) may require 6 months or longer.

SUMMARY

The indications and technique for tibial tuberosity AMZ are well described in the literature. The technique usually yields excellent results in the appropriate patient population, but the surgery has substantial potential morbidity and requires a prolonged postoperative recovery period. Most clinicians agree that patients should be restricted to partial weight bearing during the first 6 to 8 weeks after surgery to minimize the risk of tibial fracture. A formal written rehabilitation protocol that addresses the major issues of weight bearing, pain, range of motion, strength, proprioception, cardiovascular fitness, and return to sports can help organize the process and ease the communication among physicians, therapists, and the patient. Timelines for major events, such as return to full weight bearing, initiation of a running program, and return to sports activities, can be defined to help provide realistic expectations for the patient and therapist. However, the protocol should also provide for flexibility because of the variability in patients' resources and ultimate goals. The authors have found that by incorporating the important rehabilitation principles into a concise and logical protocol, most patients are able to recover successfully from AMZ surgery and return to their previous levels of activity.

REFERENCES

1. Ferguson AB Jr, Brown TD, Fu FH, et al. Relief of patellofemoral contact stress by anterior displacement of the tibial tubercle. J Bone Joint Surg Am 1979;61(2): 159–66.

2. Pidoriano AJ, Weinstein RN, Buuck DA, et al. Correlation of patellar articular lesions with results from anteromedial tibial tubercle transfer. Am J Sports Med 1997;25(4):533–7.
3. Cosgarea AJ, Schatzke MD, Seth AK, et al. Biomechanical analysis of flat and oblique tibial tubercle osteotomy for recurrent patellar instability. Am J Sports Med 1999;27(4):507–12.
4. Davis K, Caldwell P, Wayne J, et al. Mechanical comparison of fixation techniques for the tibial tubercle osteotomy. Clin Orthop Relat Res 2000;380:241–9.
5. Caldwell PE, Bohlen BA, Owen JR, et al. Dynamic confirmation of fixation techniques of the tibial tubercle osteotomy. Clin Orthop Relat Res 2004;424: 173–9.
6. Amis AA. Current concepts on anatomy and biomechanics of patellar stability. Sports Med Arthrosc 2007;15(2):48–56.
7. Rue JPH, Colton A, Zare SM, et al. Trochlear contact pressures after straight anteriorization of the tibial tuberosity. Am J Sports Med 2008;36(10):1953–9.
8. Fulkerson JP. Operative management of patellofemoral pain. Ann Chir Gynaecol 1991;80(2):224–9.
9. Fulkerson JP. Diagnosis and treatment of patients with patellofemoral pain. Am J Sports Med 2002;30(3):447–56.
10. Shelbourne KD, Porter DA, Rozzi W. Use of a modified Elmslie-Trillat procedure to improve abnormal patellar congruence angle. Am J Sports Med 1994;22(3): 318–23.
11. Naranja RJ Jr, Reilly PJ, Kuhlman JR, et al. Long-term evaluation of the Elmslie-Trillat-Maquet procedure for patellofemoral dysfunction. Am J Sports Med 1996;24(6):779–84.
12. Bellemans J, Cauwenberghs F, Witvrouw E, et al. Anteromedial tibial tubercle transfer in patients with chronic anterior knee pain and a subluxation-type patellar malalignment. Am J Sports Med 1997;25(3):375–81.
13. Garth WP Jr, DiChristina DG, Holt G. Delayed proximal repair and distal realignment after patellar dislocation. Clin Orthop Relat Res 2000;377:132–44.
14. Servien E, Verdonk PC, Neyret P. Tibial tuberosity transfer for episodic patellar dislocation. Sports Med Arthrosc 2007;15(2):61–7.
15. Ebinger TP, Boezaart A, Albright JP. Modifications of the Fulkerson osteotomy: a pilot study assessment of a novel technique of dynamic intraoperative determination of the adequacy of tubercle transfer. Iowa Orthop J 2007;27:61–4.
16. Trillat A, Dejour H, Couette A. Diagnostic et traitement des subluxations recidivantes de la rotule [Diagnosis and treatment of recurrent dislocations of the patella]. Rev Chir Orthop Reparatrice Appar Mot 1964;50(6):813–24 [in French].
17. Maquet P. Advancement of the tibial tuberosity. Clin Orthop Relat Res 1976;115: 225–30.
18. Fulkerson JP. Anteromedialization of the tibial tuberosity for patellofemoral malalignment. Clin Orthop Relat Res 1983;177:176–81.
19. Brown DE, Alexander AH, Lichtman DM. The Elmslie-Trillat procedure: evaluation in patellar dislocation and subluxation. Am J Sports Med 1984;12(2):104–8 [discussion: 109].
20. Godde S, Rupp S, Dienst M, et al. Fracture of the proximal tibia six months after Fulkerson osteotomy. A report of two cases. J Bone Joint Surg Br 2001;83(6): 832–3.
21. Stetson WB, Friedman MJ, Fulkerson JP, et al. Fracture of the proximal tibia with immediate weightbearing after a Fulkerson osteotomy. Am J Sports Med 1997; 25(4):570–4.

22. Fulkerson JP. Fracture of the proximal tibia after Fulkerson anteromedial tibial tubercle transfer. A report of four cases [letter]. Am J Sports Med 1999;27(2):265.
23. Cosgarea AJ, Freedman JA, McFarland EG. Nonunion of the tibial tubercle shingle following Fulkerson osteotomy. Am J Knee Surg 2001;14(1):51–4.
24. Eager MR, Bader DA, Kelly JD IV, et al. Delayed fracture of the tibia following anteromedialization osteotomy of the tibial tubercle. A report of 5 cases. Am J Sports Med 2004;32(4):1041–8.

Rehabilitation Following Turf Toe Injury and Plantar Plate Repair

Jeremy J. McCormick, MD[a,*], Robert B. Anderson, MD[b]

KEYWORDS

• Turf toe • Rehabilitation • Plantar plate repair • Hallux • Injury

By definition, a turf toe injury is primarily a hyperextension moment to the hallux metatarsophalangeal (MTP) joint. It was originally described by Bowers and Martin[1] in 1976 when they noted an average of 5.4 turf toe injuries per season among football players at the University of West Virginia. Similar incidences were published by Coker and colleagues[2] at the University of Arkansas and Clanton and colleagues[3] at Rice University who found 6.0 and 4.5 turf toe injuries per football season, respectively. In a survey of 80 National Football League (NFL) players, Rodeo and colleagues[4] found that 45% of active players had suffered a turf toe injury in their professional career, with 83% occurring on artificial turf.

The typical mechanism of turf toe injuries is delivery of an axial load to a foot positioned in fixed equinus. As the foot progresses into dorsiflexion, the load drives the hallux MTP into hyperextension, leading to attenuation or disruption of the plantar joint complex (**Fig. 1**). Depending on the force of impact, a spectrum of injuries can occur ranging from strain or sprain of the plantar capsular structures to frank dorsal dislocation of the toe. In addition, variants of the classic hyperextension injury can occur based on the position of the hallux and the direction of the force of injury. The most common variant involves a valgus directed force that results in greater injury to the medial and plantar-medial ligamentous structures and the tibial sesamoid complex. This injury pattern may lead to a traumatic hallux valgus deformity (**Fig. 2**).[5–7]

Classically, the injury occurs in football players participating on artificial surfaces. Recently, there has been an apparent increase in the occurrence of turf toe, with injuries occurring in nearly any field sport and on any surface. The reason for this increase is likely multifactorial, with evolution of shoewear to light-weight, flexible

[a] Department of Orthopaedic Surgery, Foot and Ankle Surgery, Washington University, 14532 South Outer Forty Drive, Chesterfield, St Louis, MO 63017, USA
[b] OrthoCarolina Foot and Ankle Institute, 250 North Caswell St @ Mercy Hospital, Suite B, Charlotte, NC 28207, USA
* Corresponding author.
E-mail address: mccormickj@wudosis.wustl.edu (J.J. McCormick).

Clin Sports Med 29 (2010) 313–323
doi:10.1016/j.csm.2009.12.010 sportsmed.theclinics.com

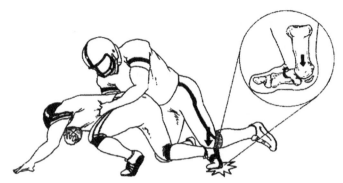

Fig. 1. Foot in fixed equinus with axially directed load leading to turf toe injury. (*Courtesy of* Michael W. Bowman, MD.)

shoes with little support, increasing numbers of sports venues using artificial turf, and changes in surface-cleat interaction all contributing in some measure.

As turf toe becomes a more recognized entity, medical care is improving as physicians and trainers are learning more about the treatment of varying grades of injury. However, it is critical to educate the medical personnel who will play a vital role in rehabilitation of the athlete back to preinjury level of competition and performance. This article reviews important concepts in the treatment of turf toe injury, with a focus on postoperative rehabilitation. To build a solid framework for this, the article also covers the pertinent anatomy of the hallux MTP joint and the evaluation of the patient with turf toe injury.

ANATOMY

Most of the stability of the hallux MTP joint comes from the capsular ligamentous sesamoid complex. Fan-shaped medial and lateral collateral ligaments course between the proximal phalanx and the metatarsal. These collateral ligaments are

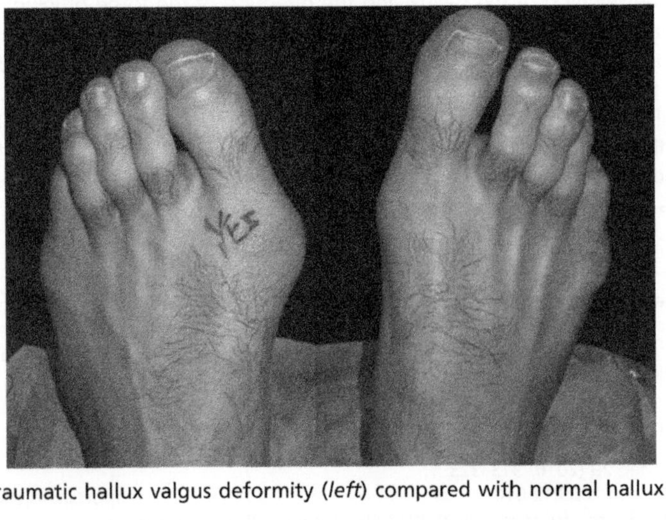

Fig. 2. A traumatic hallux valgus deformity (*left*) compared with normal hallux alignment (*right*).

important for MTP joint stability in cutting activities. The plantar plate is a separate structure that courses through the joint capsule from a firm attachment on the proximal phalanx to a weaker attachment on the metatarsal head. In addition to the collateral ligaments and the plantar plate, the abductor hallucis, adductor hallucis, and flexor hallucis brevis (FHB) all contribute to the stability and function of the capsular ligamentous complex at the hallux MTP joint (**Fig. 3**).

The FHB muscle courses on the plantar aspect of the foot and divides into a medial and lateral tendon at the level of the MTP joint. These tendons envelop the medial (tibial) and lateral (fibular) sesamoids, respectively, which provides a mechanical advantage to the FHB by elevating the metatarsal head. The sesamoids also help protect the flexor hallucis longus (FHL) as it courses along the plantar aspect of the great toe. The FHB tendon inserts at the base of the proximal phalanx with the thick volar (plantar) plate.

The capsular ligamentous complex of the hallux MTP must withstand 40% to 60% of body weight during normal gait.[8] This increases to 200% to 300% of body weight with athletic activity, and, with a running jump, the forces at the MTP joint complex can reach 800% of body weight.[9] With this in mind, it becomes clear that the capsular

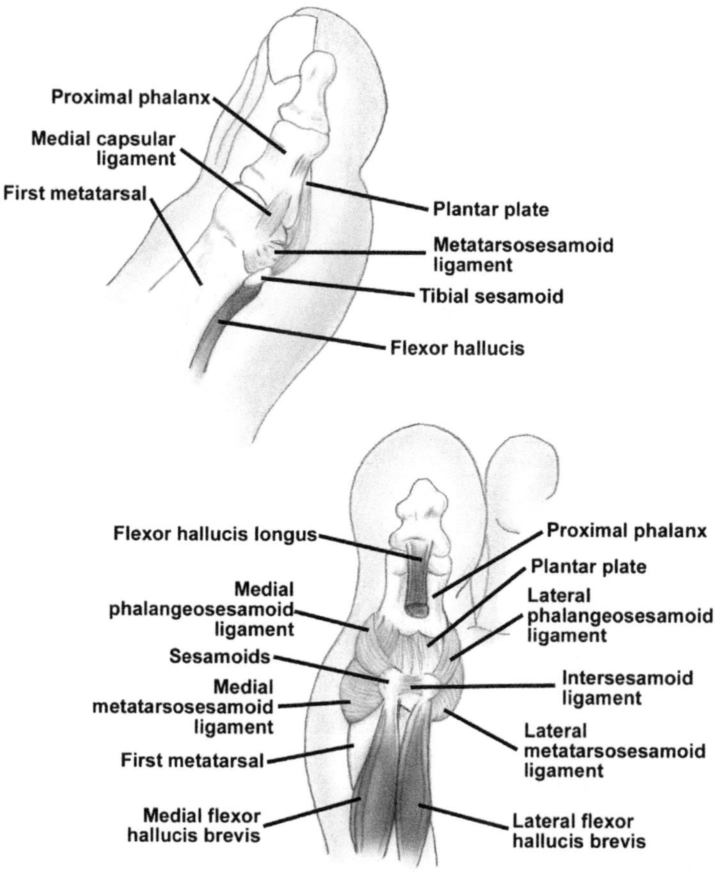

Fig. 3. Plantar view of the normal hallux MTP joint. (Available at: http://emedicine.medscape.com/article/1236962-media.)

ligamentous sesamoid complex is critical to the function of an athlete. Furthermore, it is helpful to have a working knowledge of the anatomy and mechanics of the joint to direct more careful consideration to therapeutic exercise in rehabilitation of a turf toe injury. As it might with a rotator cuff injury or knee ligament reconstruction, understanding the location and function of injured or repaired structures can only help therapists and trainers in their efforts.

EVALUATION

A turf toe injury can range from attenuation or strain of the plantar plate to frank dislocation of the MTP joint. Diagnosis of the injury can be challenging, as physical examination findings might be subtle. The most important step in properly identifying the injury is to maintain a heightened index of suspicion in a patient presenting with hallux MTP pain and swelling following an acute incident. Although the focus of this article is on rehabilitation of the turf toe injury, one must be able to properly grade the injury to define an appropriate treatment algorithm and outline accurate expectations for the athlete regarding return to play (**Table 1**).

The assessment should begin with observation of the hallux for ecchymosis or swelling. Observation should be followed by careful systematic palpation of the capsular ligamentous structures, namely the collateral ligaments, dorsal capsule, and plantar sesamoid complex. Localizing pain can be critical to diagnosis, treatment, and prognosis. For example, tenderness or pain proximal to the sesamoids suggests a strain of the musculotendinous junction of the FHB and not an unstable turf toe injury, which typically occurs distal to the sesamoids. A patient, therefore, could be afforded quicker return to play and overall better prognosis based on the findings of a careful physical examination.

The MTP joint should then be trialed through a series of range-of-motion maneuvers to evaluate stability. These maneuvers include varus and valgus stress to assess the collateral ligaments and a dorsoplantar drawer test to evaluate the plantar plate. Serial

Table 1
Summary of turf toe grading and treatment

Grade	Description/Findings	Treatment	Return to Play
I	Attenuation of plantar structures Localized swelling Minimal ecchymosis	Symptomatic	Return as tolerated
II	Partial tear of plantar structures Moderate swelling Restricted motion due to pain	Walking boot Crutches as needed	Up to 2 wk May need taping on return to play
III	Complete disruption of plantar structures Significant swelling/ ecchymosis Hallux flexion weakness Frank instability of hallux MTP	Long-term immobilization in boot or cast OR Surgical reconstruction	6–10 wk depending on sport and position Likely need taping on return to play

Adapted from Anderson RB, Shawen SB. Great-toe disorders. In: Porter DA, Schon LC, editors. Baxter's the foot and ankle in sport. 2nd edition. Philadelphia: Elsevier Health Sciences; 2007. p. 411–33.

examinations may be important, particularly in the active athlete, as the turf toe injury can progress, most commonly into valgus with a more medially based injury. Next, active flexion and extension of the MTP joint should be evaluated to determine the integrity of the flexor and extensor tendons. Grading the strength of active flexion can be helpful in deciding the extent of the injury. A decrease in flexion strength at the hallux may suggest a disruption of the FHB or plantar plate. However, the assessment of an acutely injured athlete can be difficult due to the discomfort of the injury.

Once the physical examination is completed, imaging studies are often obtained as a helpful adjunct in evaluation. Weight-bearing anteroposterior and lateral radiographs and a sesamoid axial view should be obtained. The radiographs will usually be normal. A small fleck of bone might be found from the proximal phalanx or the sesamoid, suggesting a capsular disruption. Comparison radiographs of the contralateral foot are mandatory as patients with a rupture of the plantar plate will have proximal migration of 1 or both sesamoids (**Fig. 4**).[10]

If there is clinical suspicion of a plantar plate injury, a forced dorsiflexion lateral radiograph should be obtained. With a complete disruption of the MTP joint complex, the sesamoids will not track distally with hallux MTP extension. This condition can be further demonstrated by live fluoroscopy, if available. A real-time view of the hallux MTP joint can help evaluate the sesamoids and joint complex through dynamic motion and allow comparison with the contralateral side. Much as with a dorsiflexion lateral radiograph, lack of distal sesamoid excursion with toe extension suggests a plantar soft-tissue disruption. In our practice, live fluoroscopy has become a standard part of the diagnostic algorithm and a patient education tool.

In addition to plain radiographs and fluoroscopy, magnetic resonance imaging (MRI) can be used to help identify soft-tissue injury and osseous or articular damage. T2 weighted images in multiple planes provide an optimum level of detail and will identify subtle injuries (**Fig. 5**).[11] An MRI scan should be obtained for all grade II or III injuries, as it provides critical information to help formulate a treatment plan and prognosis for the patient.

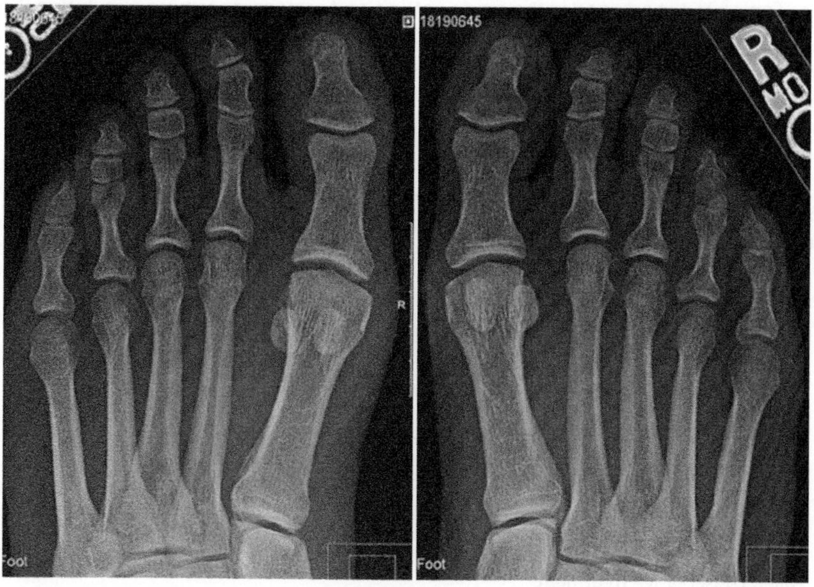

Fig. 4. Sesamoid retraction (*left*) compared with normal sesamoid position (*right*).

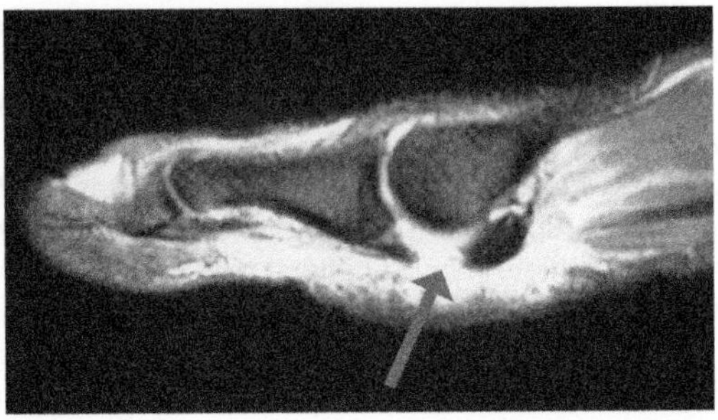

Fig. 5. T2 sagittal spectral presaturation with inversion recovery sequence MRI of the great toe. Arrow demonstrates rupture of the capsular ligamentous complex just distal to the medial sesamoid bone.

TREATMENT

As outlined earlier, treatment of turf toe depends largely on the grade of injury. Once identified, many grade I, and essentially all grade II and grade III, injuries should be referred to a foot and ankle specialist for definitive treatment. In most cases, a turf toe can be treated nonoperatively, but, for a defined set of indications, surgical repair is considered (**Box 1**). In all cases, acute and chronic, diligent rehabilitation with the assistance of a therapist or trainer is critical to the full recovery of the patient.

Nonoperative Treatment

Treatment in the early stages of all grades of injury is similar. The basic principles of rest, ice, compression, and elevation (RICE) can be applied to help reduce initial swelling. In addition, antiinflammatory medication can be used to help relieve symptoms. Taping is not advised in the acute setting as it may compromise circulation. Early on, athletes may benefit from the use of a walking boot or short leg cast with toe spica extension in slight plantarflexion. The position of splinting helps protect the hallux from extension at the MTP joint while opposing the ruptured soft-tissue structures for healing. With this protection in place, the patient may weight bear as tolerated.

Box 1
Surgical indications for turf toe injury

1. Large capsular avulsion with unstable joint
2. Diastasis of bipartite sesamoid
3. Diastasis of sesamoid fracture
4. Retraction of sesamoid(s)
5. Traumatic hallux valgus deformity
6. Vertical instability (positive Lachman test)
7. Loose body
8. Chondral injury
9. Failed conservative treatment

Grade I injury, or attenuation of the plantar structures of the MTP joint, allows athletes to return to competition with little or no loss of playing time. The toe may benefit from taping in slight plantarflexion to provide compression and limit motion (**Fig. 6**). In addition, athletes should modify their shoes to include stiff soles with turf toe plates to limit hallux MTP extension (**Fig. 7**). Another option is a custom orthotic device with a Morton extension. In the case of a more medially based injury, a toe separator between the hallux and second toe may provide additional support.

If symptoms permit, therapists can begin working with gentle range of motion as soon as 3 to 5 days after the injury. Initial exercise consists of passive plantarflexion to prevent sesamoid adhesions while protecting the healing soft tissues. The patient's level of discomfort will dictate the pace of early rehabilitation work. If maintaining overall endurance is important to the athlete, low-impact exercises can be attempted, as long as the toe is protected. Bicycling, elliptical training, and pool therapy are all viable options. It is important to follow the patient carefully with serial examinations as the deformity can progress with athletic activity. Cortisone or anesthetic injections are not advised.

Grade II injuries, or partial plantar capsular ligamentous rupture, will generally result in loss of playing time of at least 2 weeks. These injuries are treated with a similar regimen used for grade I injuries. Again, gentle range of motion can begin as early as 3 to 5 days, if symptoms permit. As long as the toe is protected with a boot or toe spica taping, low-impact exercises can be attempted. The athlete should not participate in explosive, push-off activities until low-impact exercise and jogging is tolerated without pain or limitation. Also, the requirements of an athlete's sport or position will play a role in their ability to return to play, as an offensive lineman in football can tolerate a splinted, stiff great toe much more easily than a defensive back. As with grade I injuries, shoewear should be adjusted to include a stiff sole and turf toe plate. Ultimately, return to play will be dictated by the athlete's symptoms and their ability to reach near preinjury level of performance.

Grade III injury, or complete plantar capsular ligamentous rupture, may require up to 8 weeks of recovery. With these injuries, a longer period of immobilization is appropriate before return to play. Again, return will be dictated by symptoms. Ideally, the hallux MTP will have 50 to 60 degrees of painless passive dorsiflexion before running or explosive activities are attempted. As with grade II injuries, the athlete's sport or position will play a role in return to play and should be considered carefully. It must

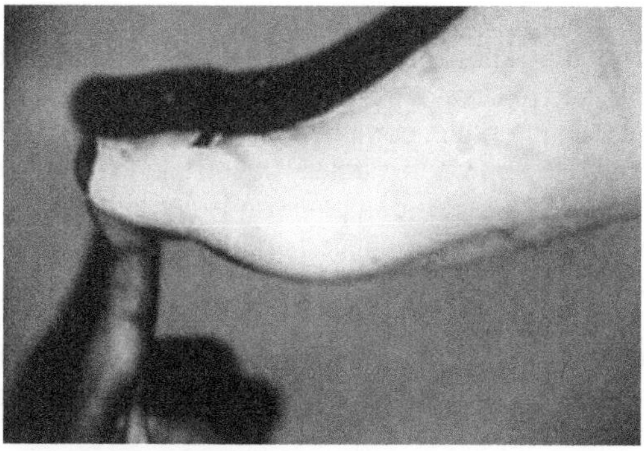

Fig. 6. Turf toe taping. Finger is applying plantar pressure to demonstrate limitation of hallux dorsiflexion due to taping.

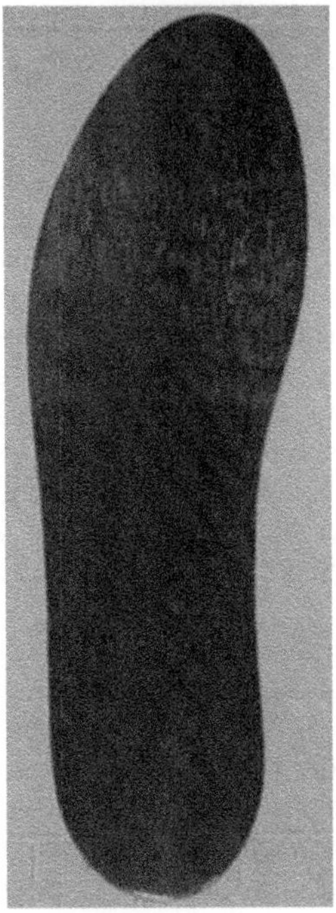

Fig. 7. Example of a carbon-fiber turf toe plate.

be made clear to the athlete that a recovery period of up to 6 months can be expected before complete resolution of symptoms where shoewear modifications and taping are not necessary.

Surgical Treatment

Operative treatment of a turf toe injury is seldom necessary. The decision to treat a patient surgically can be difficult and is based on the indications outlined in **Box 1**. In addition to acute injury, one must consider surgical intervention if patients fail conservative measures and remain unable to perform to their capabilities, such as with loss of push-off strength. Because of the infrequency with which these injuries are surgically repaired, they should always be referred to a foot and ankle specialist.

The goal of surgery is to restore normal anatomy to regain the stability and function of the plantar capsular ligamentous complex of the hallux MTP joint. A classic medial "J" type is typically used to approach medially based injuries, and a dual incision technique has been described to repair complete capsular ligamentous rupture (**Fig. 8**). Once the soft-tissue structures are identified and the injury is defined, the soft-tissue repair is completed.[7,12]

If all that is found is a capsular disruption, typically distal to the sesamoids, then the soft tissues are directly sutured to one another, end to end. If the injury is solely a medially based injury (traumatic hallux valgus) then a percutaneous adductor tenotomy should be performed in addition to the medial soft-tissue repair. This tenotomy helps to balance the soft-tissue structures of the capsular ligamentous complex, and reduces valgus deforming forces at the hallux MTP joint. In addition, in this scenario,

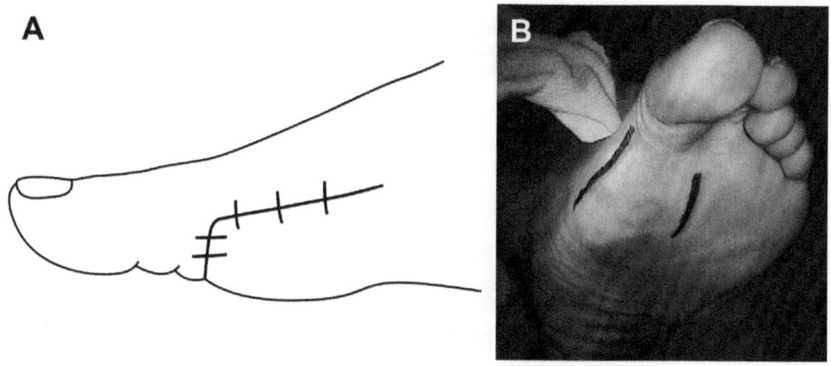

Fig. 8. (*A*) Classic medial "J" incision. (*B*) Dual incision.

the medial eminence of the metatarsal head is resected to allow for capsulodesis, as with a standard bunion procedure.

If there is a sesamoid fracture, or diastasis of a bipartite sesamoid, the authors recommend attempting to preserve 1 pole of the sesamoid, if possible. Ideally a smaller distal pole is amenable to excision. The soft tissues are then repaired by passing a suture through a drill hole in the sesamoid. If a complete sesamoidectomy is required, then the authors recommend detaching the abductor hallucis tendon from its distal insertion and transferring it plantarly into the soft-tissue defect left by the excised sesamoids (**Fig. 9**). This should improve the plantar restraint to dorsiflexion forces, augment the flexion power of the hallux MTP, and provide healthy collagen to the site of injury.

Postoperative Management

The postoperative management of surgical reconstruction of the turf toe is challenging because of the need for balancing soft-tissue protection with early range of motion. Careful monitoring and assistance from a physical therapist or athletic trainer is paramount. Immediately after surgery, a toe spica splint should be used to keep the toe in 5 to 10 degrees of plantarflexion (**Fig. 10**). In the case of traumatic hallux valgus, the toe

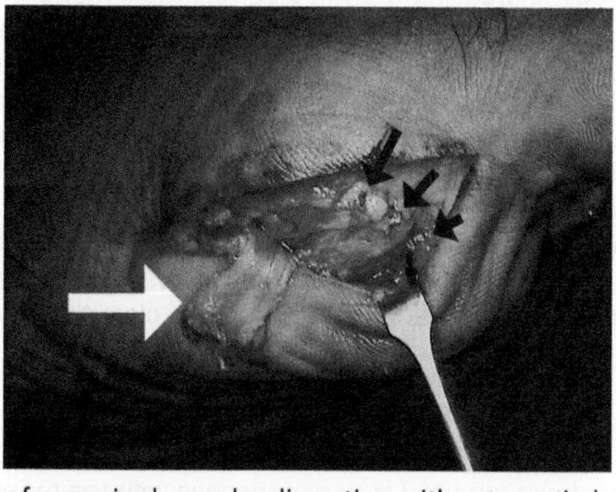

Fig. 9. Medial view of a repaired capsular disruption with sutures tied. Large arrow on left points to abductor hallucis tendon to be used in transfer. Three smaller arrows on right point to tied knots.

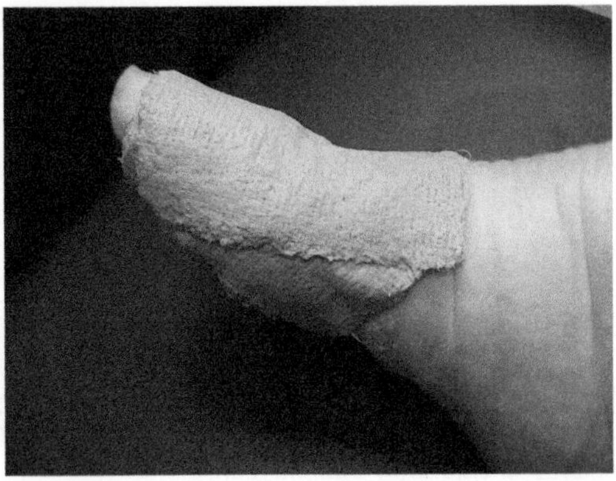

Fig. 10. Postoperative toe spica splint in 5 to 10 degrees of plantarflexion at the hallux MTP joint.

should also be maintained in slight varus to protect the repair. Under careful supervision, gentle passive range of motion can be initiated at 5 to 7 days to minimize the development of arthrofibrosis at the sesamoid-metatarsal articulation. Care should be taken to avoid excessive dorsiflexion and jeopardize the surgical reconstruction.

The patient should remain non–weight bearing for 4 weeks with a removable splint or protective boot. Slight varus overcorrection of the traumatic hallux valgus repair can be maintained with taping, the use of a toe separator, or soft-tissue regulator. At night the patient should wear a removable bunion splint with plantar restraint.

At 4 weeks, the patient may begin protected weight bearing in a boot. At this point active motion of the hallux MTP joint can be initiated. Progression will be dictated by the athletes and their symptoms. As the patient is only allowed protected weight bearing, high-impact running activities should obviously be avoided at this stage. Pool therapy can be attempted with a water level up to the mid-chest to help unload the foot and surgically repaired toe as the athlete attempts gentle weight bearing and gait.

At 8 weeks, the patient will discontinue the use of the boot and transition to a stiff-sole shoe modified with a turf toe plate to prevent hallux MTP hyperextension. The athlete may now begin increasing activities as tolerated with protective taping and shoewear. Gradually, progression can be made from low-impact activities, such as bicycling, to medium-impact activities, such as elliptical training. Once the athlete is comfortable with this, advancement can be made to light jogging and then straight-line running. The athlete should begin cutting and jumping activities only after being able to regain the ability to straight-ahead sprint without pain.

In our experience, a contact athlete is able to return to full activity by 16 weeks. It is important to outline appropriate expectations for recovery, particularly with high-level athletes who are driven to return to their preinjury level of performance as soon as possible. Despite a return to full activity, it should be clear that it will take at least 6 months, and often as long as 12 months, to obtain a full recovery.

SURGICAL OUTCOMES

Various investigators have reported their experiences with turf toe injuries. Anderson[7] reported on 19 high-level athletes who underwent evaluation for disabling turf toe injuries. Nine required operative repair. All but 2 patients returned to full athletic activity with documented restoration of plantar stability. There were no operative complications. Coker and colleagues[13] reported on 9 athletes with hyperextension injury to the first MTP joint, finding that the most common long-term complaints were joint stiffness and pain with athletic activity. Clanton and colleagues[3] had a larger group of 20 patients at a 5-year follow-up from turf toe injury. He reported that 50% of these athletes had persisting symptoms of pain and stiffness.

SUMMARY

The evaluation and diagnosis of turf toe injuries is improving as it becomes a more recognized pattern of injury to the hallux MTP joint. With an understanding of the anatomy of the injury and the ability to focus on important diagnostic and radiographic clues, turf toe can be diagnosed, assessed, and treated accurately, with surgical repair when indicated. Regardless of the grade of injury, rehabilitation of the athlete under the guidance of a physical therapist or athletic trainer is critical to complete recovery. With appropriate care, athletes can successfully return to play and efficiently reach their preinjury level of participation.

REFERENCES

1. Bowers KD Jr, Martin RB. Turf-toe: a shoe-surface related football injury. Med Sci Sports 1976;8(2):81–3.
2. Coker TP, Arnold JA, Weber DL. Traumatic lesions of the metatarsophalangeal joint of the great toe in athletes. J Ark Med Soc 1978;74(8):309–17.
3. Clanton TO, Butler JE, Eggert A. Injuries to the metatarsophalangeal joints in athletes. Foot Ankle 1986;7(3):162–76.
4. Rodeo SA, O'Brien S, Warren RF, et al. Turf-toe: an analysis of metatarsophalangeal joint sprains in professional football players. Am J Sports Med 1990;18(3):280–5.
5. Watson TS, Anderson RB, Davis WH. Periarticular injuries to the hallux metatarsophalangeal joint in athletes. Foot Ankle Clin 2000;5(3):687–713.
6. Douglas DP, Davidson DM, Robinson JE, et al. Rupture of the medial collateral ligament of the first metatarsophalangeal joint in a professional soccer player. J Foot Ankle Surg 1997;36(5):388–90.
7. Anderson RB. Turf toe injuries of the hallux metatarsophalangeal joint. Tech Foot Ankle Surg 2002;1(2):102–11.
8. Stokes IA, Hutton WC, Stott JR, et al. Forces under the hallux valgus foot before and after surgery. Clin Orthop Relat Res 1979;142:64–72.
9. Nigg BM. Biomechanical aspects of running. In: Nigg BM, editor. Biomechanics of running shoes. Champaign (IL): Human Kinetics Publishers; 1986. p. 1–25.
10. Prieskorn D, Graves SC, Smith RA. Morphometric analysis of the plantar plate apparatus of the first metatarsophalangeal joint. Foot Ankle 1993;14(4):204–7.
11. Tewes DP, Fischer DA, Fritts HM, et al. MRI findings of acute turf toe. A case report and review of anatomy. Clin Orthop Relat Res 1994;304:200–3.
12. McCormick JJ, Anderson RB. The great toe: failed turf toe, chronic turf toe, and complicated sesamoids injuries. Foot Ankle Clin 2009;14(2):135–50.
13. Coker TP, Arnold JA, Weber DL. Traumatic lesions of the metatarsophalangeal joint of the great toe in athletes. Am J Sports Med 1978;6(6):326–34.

Index

Note: Page numbers of article titles are in **boldface** type.

Clin Sports Med 29 (2010) 325–330
doi:10.1016/S0278-5919(10)00010-4

O

P

Q

R

S

T

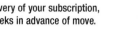